Registration Exam Questions IV

Nadia Bukhari (Series Managing Editor)

BPharm (Hons), MRPharmS, PG Dip (Pharm Prac), PG Dip (T&L in Higher Ed), FHEA
Senior Teaching Fellow and Pre-registration Co-ordinator, UCL School of Pharmacy, London, UK and Chairwoman, Pre-registration Conferences, Royal Pharmaceutical Society

Oksana Pyzik (Assistant Editor)

MPharmS
Teaching Fellow, Department of Practice and Policy, UCL School of Pharmacy, London, UK

Ryan Hamilton (Contributor)

MRPharmS
Clinical pharmacist, University Hospitals of Leicester NHS Trust, and active member of the UK Clinical Pharmacy Association's infection network

Amar Iqbal (Contributor)

MPharm (Hons), MRPharmS, PgDip (Clin Pharm)
Pre-registration and Student Support Lead, Birmingham and Solihull Local Practice Forum

Alistair Murray (Contributor)

MPharm (Hons), MRPharmS, Independent Prescriber
Clinical Lead, Green Light Pharmacy
Honorary Lecturer, University of Nottingham and UCL School of Pharmacy

PP
Ph
Pharmaceutical Press

Published by the Pharmaceutical Press

1 Lambeth High Street, London SE1 7JN, UK

© Pharmaceutical Press 2015

(**PP**) is a trade mark of Pharmaceutical Press

Pharmaceutical Press is the publishing division of the Royal Pharmaceutical Society

First published 2015   l O o7&/ I ᐳS 6

Typeset by Laserwords Private Limited, Chennai, India
Printed in Great Britain by TJ International, Padstow, Cornwall

ISBN 978 0 85711 155 5

Disclaimer

The views expressed in this book are solely those of the author and do not necessarily reflect the views or policies of the Royal Pharmaceutical Society. This book does NOT guarantee success in the registration exam but can be used as an aid for revision.

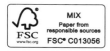

MIX
Paper from
responsible sources
FSC   FSC® C013056
www.fsc.org

I would like to dedicate this book to my family. Without their continued support I wouldn't be the woman I am today – Nadia Bukhari.

Contents

Preface   *ix*
Acknowledgements   xi
About the authors   xiii
Abbreviations   xvii
How to use this book   xxi

Open book questions	**1**
Simple completion questions	1
Multiple completion questions	16
Classification questions	26
Statement questions	31
Closed book questions	**43**
Simple completion questions	43
Multiple completion questions	59
Classification questions	71
Statement questions	78
Calculation questions	**89**
Simple completion questions	89
Multiple completion questions	108
Classification questions	111
Statement questions	114

Answers

Open book answers   **117**

Closed book answers   **145**

Calculation answers   **167**

Index   185

Preface

After the success of the first three editions of *Registration Exam Questions*, a decision was made to write a fourth book testing all the main aspects of the registration examination.

This book is a bank of over 500 questions, which are similar to the style of the registration examination. The questions are based on law and ethics, and clinical pharmacy and therapeutic aspects of the registration examination syllabus, as well as pharmaceutical calculations.

After completing four years of study and graduating with a Master of Pharmacy (MPharm) degree, graduates are required to undertake training as a pre-registration pharmacist before they can sit the registration examination.

Pre-registration training is the period of employment on which graduates must embark and effectively complete before they can register as a pharmacist in Great Britain. In most cases it is a one-year period following the pharmacy degree; for sandwich course students it is integrated within the undergraduate programme.

On successfully passing the registration examination, pharmacy graduates can register as a pharmacist in Great Britain.

The registration examination harmonises the testing of skills in practice during the pre-registration year. It tests:

- knowledge
- the application of knowledge
- calculation
- time management
- managing stress
- comprehension
- recall
- interpretation
- evaluation

There are two examination papers: an open book and a closed book paper. Questions are based on practice-based situations and are designed to test the thinking and knowledge that lie behind any action.

EXAMINATION FORMAT

The registration examination consists of two papers:

1   closed book (no reference material can be used): 90 questions in 90 minutes (1.5 hours)
2   open book (two specified reference sources permitted):

- 80 questions in 150 minutes (2.5 hours)
- 60 non-calculation-style (recommended time for these 1.5 hours)
- 20 calculation-style (recommended time 1 hour).

The calculation-style questions are grouped together as a section of the paper.

The reference sources that the General Pharmaceutical Council permit for the registration examination are:

- *British National Formulary*
- *BNF for Children*

The registration examination is crucial for pharmacy graduates wishing to register in Great Britain.

Due to student demand, the *Registration Exam Questions* series will become an annual publication, with brand new questions written on all aspects of the examination. Any updates to the examination will be taken into consideration.

Preparation is the key. This book cannot guarantee that you pass the registration examination; however, it can help you to practise the clinical pharmacy, pharmaceutical calculations, and law and ethics questions, all very important aspects of the registration examination, and, as they say, 'practice makes perfect'.

Good luck with the examination.

Nadia Bukhari
February 2015

Acknowledgements

The editor wishes to acknowledge the support from students and colleagues at the UCL School of Pharmacy. Thank you to all four contributors – Ryan Hamilton, Oksana Pyzik, Amar Iqbal, and Alistair Murray.

Nadia Bukhari would like to express thanks to our editors at Pharmaceutical Press for their support and patience in the writing of this book, and especially to Christina Karaviotis and Erasmis Kidd, for their guidance.

About the authors

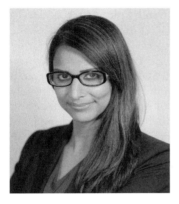

Nadia Bukhari is the Chair for the RPS Pre-registration conferences. She developed the extremely popular and over-subscribed conference, when it first started in 2012. Nadia graduated from the School of Pharmacy, University of London, in 1999. After qualifying, she worked as a pharmacy manager at Westbury Chemist, Streatham, for a year, after which she moved on to work for Bart's and the London NHS Trust as a clinical pharmacist in surgery. It was at this time that Nadia developed an interest in teaching, as part of her role involved the responsibility of being a teacher practitioner for the School of Pharmacy, University of London. Two and a half years later, she commenced working for the School of Pharmacy, University of London, as the pre-registration co-ordinator and the academic facilitator. This position involved teaching therapeutics to Master of Pharmacy students and assisting the director of undergraduate studies.

While teaching undergraduate students, Nadia completed her Post Graduate Diploma in Pharmacy Practice and her Post Graduate Diploma in Teaching in Higher Education. She then took on the role of the Master of Pharmacy Programme Manager, which involved the management of the undergraduate degree as well as being the pre-registration coordinator for the university.

Since the merger with UCL, Nadia has now taken on the role of Senior Teaching Fellow and Pre-registration Coordinator for the university. She has a diploma in professional counselling and is a fellow of the Higher Education Academy. Nadia has recently taken on the responsibility of the course coordinator for the final year of the MPharm.

Nadia will be leading the Professional Leadership module at UCL SoP, which involves designing, teaching and implementing the course to all four-year students studying the MPharm course. This module ties in well with Nadia's proposed PhD thesis on 'Professional Leadership in Pharmacy Education'.

Nadia has many responsibilities within the professional body, the Royal Pharmaceutical Society. She is chairwoman for the pre-registration conferences and is lead pharmacist for the foundation programme development.

Nadia's interest in writing emerged in her first year of working in academia. Nine years on, Nadia has authored six titles with the Pharmaceutical Press. She is currently writing her seventh title, which is due to publish in February 2016. Nadia is also an MCQ question writer for the ONtrackpharmacy.com. Nadia's 12 years of experience as a pre-registration coordinator and clinical lecturer, coupled with the fact that she was a question writer for the registration exam for the RPSGB for four years, ignited her interest in private coaching for the examination. She has privately tutored many students, all of whom have given her positive feedback and have passed their exams in the first attempt after receiving coaching from her. For more information please visit her website: www.preregtuition.co.uk

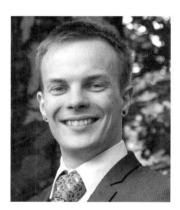

Ryan Hamilton is a clinical pharmacist at University Hospitals of Leicester NHS Trust and an active member of the UK Clinical Pharmacy Association's infection network. He also sits on the Royal Pharmaceutical Society's Education Expert Advisory Panel and was previously the president of the British Pharmaceutical Students' Association (2011-2012).

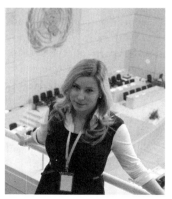

Oksana Pyzik is currently working as a Teaching Fellow at the UCL School of Pharmacy in the Department of Practice and Policy. She has also worked for the Royal Pharmaceutical Society as the Foundation Programme Lead Pharmacist and is part of the RPS Pre-registration Teaching Panel. Her research interests lie in Global Health and Public Health and she is a Champion for the UCL Global Citizenship Programme, acting as the International Student Advisor. Oksana also sits on the Teaching Innovation Committee and the Exam Review Board at

UCL. Previously, Oksana has worked as a locum in community pharmacies and was the Lead Pharmacist Researcher for a joint project between the International Pharmaceutical Federation (FIP) and the International Pharmaceutical Students' Federation, and the European Law Students' Association, on international competition law and public health.

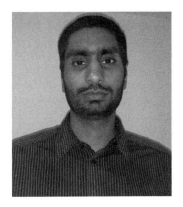 After graduating with first class honours from Aston University in 2007, **Amar Iqbal** undertook his pre-registration year with Alliance Boots in a busy community pharmacy in Warwickshire. Amar's skills were quickly recognised and upon qualification in 2008 he went on to become store manager at the UK's first ever hospital outpatient pharmacy collaboration. It was in this role that Amar personally started his Postgraduate Clinical Diploma in 2009, which he went on to complete upon switching to the National Health Service in 2010.

Within the NHS, Amar has covered specialties including medicines information, medicines admissions, gastroenterology, neuro-rehabilitation, ophthalmology, and surgery while at Sandwell and West Birmingham Hospitals NHS Trust. Currently, Amar is specialising in women's and children's healthcare, serving as a Senior Clinical Pharmacist and Teacher Practitioner at the Heart of England NHS Foundation Teaching Trust. Here, he is involved in policy and formulary writing, reviewing financial reports, as well as being closely involved in inducting, training and educating healthcare professionals. Amar also works closely with Aston University on student placements and examination assessments among others.

Amar is a keen advocate of the Royal Pharmaceutical Society (RPS) and has a dedicated role as Pre-registration and Student Support Lead at Birmingham and Solihull Local Practice Forum, which was voted 'LPF of the Year' at the RPS Awards (2012). He also sits on the RPS Pre-registration Advisory Panel helping to provide support material (such as the BNF for Children Presentation and Quick Reference Guide) for upcoming pharmacists. In addition, Amar has undertaken consultancy work, produced new training material, reviewed national guidance, been a locum pharmacist, and has worked for both the RPSGB and now GPhC.

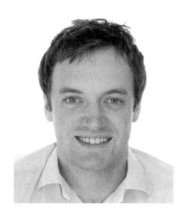

Alistair Murray is a community pharmacist who registered in 2003, originally graduating from Nottingham in 2002. He is an independent prescriber with an interest in travel medicine and unscheduled primary care. His role as Clinical Lead at Green Light Pharmacy in London includes service development, training pharmacists, pre-regs and the wider pharmacy and healthcare teams, as well as working closely with people using the pharmacy to maximise the benefit from using medicines and public health services. Alistair has been a pre-reg tutor since 2006 and has helped to develop and deliver Green Light Pharmacy's pre-reg training course, as well as contributing to the Pharmacy Live training initiative that Green Light Pharmacy runs in association with UCL. He is an honorary lecturer at the University of Nottingham and UCL School of Pharmacy. Leisure activities include travelling, sailing and skiing and also collecting art, wine and far too many house and disco 12" vinyl records.

Abbreviations

ACBS	Advisory Committee on Borderline Substances
ACE	angiotensin-converting enzyme
AV	arteriovenous
b.d.	bis die
BMI	body mass index
BNF	*British National Formulary*
Bpm	beats per minute
BSA	body surface area
CD	controlled drug
CE	*conformité européenne*
CFC	chlorofluorocarbon
CHM	Commission on Human Medicines
CHMP	Committee for Medicinal Products for Human Use
COX	cyclo-oxygenase
COPD	chronic obstructive pulmonary disease
CPD	continuing professional development
CrCl	creatinine clearance (mL/minute)
CSM	Committee on Safety of Medicines
CYT	cytochrome
DigCl	digoxin clearance (L/hour)
DMARD	disease-modifying antirheumatic drug
DNG	discount not given
DPF	*Dental Practitioners' Formulary*
EEA	European Economic Area
e/c	enteric-coated
eGFR	estimated glomerular filtration rate
EHC	emergency hormonal contraception
GP	general practitioner
G6PD	glucose-6-phosphate dehydrogenase
GPhC	General Pharmaceutical Council
GSL	general sales list
GTN	glyceryl trinitrate
HIV	human immunodeficiency virus
HRT	hormone replacement therapy
IBS	irritable bowel syndrome

IBW	ideal body weight
IDA	industrial denatured alcohol
IM	intramuscular
INR	international normalised ratio
IV	intravenous
IUD	intrauterine device
MAOI	monoamine oxidase inhibitor
MD	maximum single dose
MDD	maximum daily dose
MDI	metered-dose inhaler
MEP	*Medicines, Ethics and Practice Guide*
MHRA	Medicines and Healthcare products Regulatory Agency
MMR	measles, mumps and rubella
MR, m/r	modified release
MUPS	multiple-unit pellet system
MUR	Medicines Use Review
NHS	National Health Service
NICE	National Institute for Health and Care Excellence
NMS	New Medicines Service
NSAIDs	non-steroidal anti-inflammatory drugs
OC	oral contraceptive
o.d.	omne die (every day)
o.m.	omni mane (every morning)
o.n.	omni nocte (every night)
OP	original pack
ORT	oral rehydration therapy
OTC	over-the-counter
P	pharmacy
PAGB	Proprietary Association of Great Britain
PCT	primary care trust
PIL	patient information leaflet
PMR	patient medication record
POM	prescription-only medicine
POM-V	prescription-only medicine – veterinarian
POM-VPS	prescription-only medicine – veterinarian, pharmacist, suitably qualified person
PSA	prostate-specific antigen
PSNC	Pharmaceutical Services Negotiating Committee
q.d.s.	quarter die sumendum (to be taken four times daily)
RPS	Royal Pharmaceutical Society (formerly RPSGB)

SARSS	Suspected Adverse Reaction Surveillance Scheme
SLS	selected list scheme
SOP	standard operating procedure
SPC	Summary of Product Characteristics
SSRI	selective serotonin reuptake inhibitor
TCA	tricyclic antidepressant
TDS	three times a day
TPN	total parenteral nutrition
TSDA	trade-specific denatured alcohol
UTI	urinary tract infection
WHO	World Health Organization

How to use this book

The book is divided into two main sections: open book and closed book. There is also a brand new section which features calculation questions.

Each section has four different styles of multiple choice questions, which are also used in the registration examination: simple completion, multiple completion, classification and statements.

SIMPLE COMPLETION QUESTIONS

Each of the questions or statements in this section is followed by five suggested answers. Select the best answer in each situation.

For example:
A patient on your ward has been admitted with a gastric ulcer, which is currently being treated. She has a history of arthritis and cardiac problems. Which of her drugs is most likely to have caused the gastric ulcer?

- ☐ A   paracetamol
- ☐ B   naproxen
- ☐ C   furosemide
- ☐ D   propranolol
- ☐ E   codeine phosphate

MULTIPLE COMPLETION QUESTIONS

Each one of the questions or incomplete statements in this section is followed by three responses. For each question, one or more of the responses is/are correct. Decide which of the responses is/are correct, then choose:

A   if 1, 2 and 3 are correct
B   if 1 and 2 only are correct

C   if 2 and 3 only are correct
D   if 1 only is correct
E   if 3 only is correct

For example:
A patient presents an FP10D to you.
Which of the below *cannot* be prescribed on this type of form?

1   ciprofloxacin
2   diclofenac
3   paracetamol

CLASSIFICATION

In this section, for each numbered question, select the one lettered option that most closely corresponds to the answer. Within each group of questions each lettered option may be used once, more than once or not at all.

For example:
Which of the following vitamins:

1   can cause ocular defects in deficiency states?
2   is necessary for the production of blood-clotting factors?
3   prevents scurvy?
4   can be used for the treatment of rickets?

A   vitamin A
B   vitamin C
C   vitamin D
D   vitamin E
E   vitamin K

STATEMENTS

The questions in this section consist of a statement in the top row followed by a second statement beneath.

You need to:

decide whether the *first* statement is true or false

decide whether the *second* statement is true or false

Then choose:

A   if both statements are true and the second statement is a correct explanation of the first statement

B   if both statements are true but the second statement is not a correct explanation of the first statement

C   if the first statement is true but the second statement is false

D   if the first statement is false but the second statement is true

E   if both statements are false

For example:

First statement

Microgynon is an example of a combined oral contraceptive pill.

Second statement

Combined pills contain oestrogen and testosterone.

The closed book questions should be attempted without using any references sources, as you would for the examination.

The open book questions should be attempted with the GPhC's permitted reference sources for the registration examination, which are:

- *British National Formulary (BNF)*
- *BNF for Children*

Answers to the questions are at the end of the book. Brief explanations or a suitable reference for sourcing the answer are given, to aid understanding and to facilitate learning.

Important: This text refers to the edition of the BNF current when text was written. Please always consult the LATEST version for the most up-to-date information.

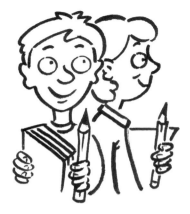

Open book questions

SIMPLE COMPLETION QUESTIONS

Amar Iqbal

Each of the questions or statements in this section is followed by five suggested answers. Select the best answer in each situation.

Questions 1–3 concern Child J, aged 12, who presents to hospital with a suspected staphylococcal skin infection. Child J has a documented history of acute porphyria.

1   Prior to prescribing any antibiotics, which of the following factors need not be considered by the prescribing doctor looking after Child J?

   ☐ A   allergy status
   ☐ B   ethnic origin
   ☐ C   formulation
   ☐ D   taking skin swabs
   ☐ E   treatment duration

2   Which of the following statements is not true regarding acute porphyria?

   ☐ A   They are hereditary disorders.
   ☐ B   They affect haem biosynthesis.
   ☐ C   Attacks are common before puberty.
   ☐ D   Attacks can be induced by certain drugs.
   ☐ E   Haem arginate can be used as a treatment.

3   On your morning ward round while you are reviewing Child J, the duty consultant asks for your advice on which of the following antibiotics is safe to prescribe for his presenting complaint. What do you advise?

☐ A   clindamycin
☐ B   erythromycin
☐ C   flucloxacillin
☐ D   griseofulvin
☐ E   rifampicin

Questions 4–5 concern the aminoglycoside antibiotic agent, gentamicin, which is widely used in your hospital trust.

4   You are in the process of updating the listed indications for intravenous use of this drug in the hospital formulary. Which one of the following is not a recognised indication for intravenous gentamicin?

☐ A   acute pyelonephritis
☐ B   bacterial endocarditis
☐ C   listerial meningitis
☐ D   neonatal sepsis
☐ E   urinary tract infection

5   Which of the following is an irreversible side-effect of gentamicin?

☐ A   antibiotic-related colitis
☐ B   electrolyte disturbances
☐ C   nephrotoxicity
☐ D   ototoxicity
☐ E   stomatitis

Questions 6–8 concern a phone call you receive from your local GP surgery for some advice regarding Mr DW, one of your regular patients who is on the following repeat medication:

Amlodipine 10 mg OM
Aspirin 75 mg OM

6   Your local GP would like to prescribe simvastatin for hypercholesterolaemia and wants to know the maximum dose that he can give to Mr
DW as his recent blood cholesterol level was at 6 mmol/L.

    ☐ A   5 mg
    ☐ B   10 mg
    ☐ C   20 mg
    ☐ D   40 mg
    ☐ E   80 mg

7   Which of the following side-effects of simvastatin does Mr DW not
need to report immediately to his GP?

    ☐ A   cough
    ☐ B   difficulty breathing
    ☐ C   headache
    ☐ D   muscle pain
    ☐ E   weight loss

8   Which of the following monitoring is needed before initiating statin
therapy in order to ensure that Mr DW's lipid abnormality is not due
to another resolvable cause?

    ☐ A   blood glucose levels
    ☐ B   creatine kinase levels
    ☐ C   liver function tests
    ☐ D   platelet counts
    ☐ E   thyroid function tests

Questions 9–12 concern a phone call you receive from a rheumatology
registrar regarding advice for Mrs RA for whom she wants to initiate
methotrexate for arthritis.

9   In which of the listed group of patients does methotrexate not need to
be used with caution?

    ☐ A   In those with acute porphyria.
    ☐ B   In those with hepatic impairment.
    ☐ C   In those with a raised neutrophil count.
    ☐ D   In women who are pregnant.
    ☐ E   In those with renal impairment.

10 Which of the following is not suitable advice for you to provide Mrs RA when counselling her on taking her newly prescribed methotrexate?

  □ A   The drug is needed to treat her arthritis.
  □ B   The drug is taken once weekly in the morning.
  □ C   The drug will be given to her in a single strength.
  □ D   The drug will be prescribed with folic acid.
  □ E   The drug does not require routine monitoring.

11 Which of the following would you advise Mrs RA as not being a sign of methotrexate-related toxicity?

  □ A   becoming easily bruised
  □ B   developing mouth ulcers
  □ C   having abdominal pain
  □ D   shortness of breath
  □ E   precipitation of diabetes

12 Which one of the following drugs can Mrs RA safely purchase over the counter for its analgesic action while she is on methotrexate?

  □ A   aspirin
  □ B   co-codamol
  □ C   diclofenac
  □ D   ibuprofen
  □ E   mefenamic acid

Questions 13–14 concern topical dermatological preparations and their use in Mr CT, a 26-year-old male, who has presented to his GP with symptoms suggestive of scabies.

13 What is the maximum recommended usual quantity of *Lyclear Dermal Cream* that can be practically dispensed to a patient who requires two applications, each a week apart, for scabies?

  □ A   30 g
  □ B   60 g
  □ C   90 g
  □ D   100 g
  □ E   120 g

14 To which of the following body parts does the manufacturer recommend you should not apply *Lyclear Dermal Cream* when treating scabies?

- ☐ A   arms
- ☐ B   ears
- ☐ C   feet
- ☐ D   legs
- ☐ E   neck

Questions 15–17 concern the use of vaccinations.

15 Child SW, who is two months old, has a history of anaphylaxis from egg-based products. Which of the following vaccines must be given to Child SW in a hospital setting under specialist referral due to evidence of previous anaphylactic reactions?

- ☐ A   *Fluarix*
- ☐ B   *Meningitec*
- ☐ C   *Pediacel*
- ☐ D   *Pneumovax* II
- ☐ E   *Rotarix*

16 Mr GT is due to travel to Africa for a safari trip in three weeks' time. He approaches you in your community pharmacy for advice regarding the oral typhoid vaccine that has been prescribed for him. He would like to know when he should have his last capsule in order to ensure that he starts his treatment in time to gain adequate protection before he gets to Africa. What should you advise?

- ☐ A   On the day of travel
- ☐ B   1 day before travel
- ☐ C   3 days before travel
- ☐ D   5 days before travel
- ☐ E   7 days before travel

17 Child FS is due for his first routine MMR vaccine. The outpatient clinic telephones you to confirm its appropriateness. Which of the following is not a contraindication for the use of the MMR vaccine?

- ☐ A   known allergy to gelatin
- ☐ B   known allergy to neomycin
- ☐ C   regular use of ciclosporin
- ☐ D   use of human normal immunoglobulin in the last ten weeks
- ☐ E   use of a live vaccine in the last eight weeks

Questions 18–19 concern the use of drugs that can affect the genito-urinary system.

18 You are covering a gynaecology ward when you are asked by the multidisciplinary team to suggest suitable hormone replacement therapy (HRT) for Mrs AC, a 55-year-old woman with an intact uterus. She has no past medical history of note, does not take any regular medications, and has no known allergies or sensitivities. Which is the most suitable preparation?

  ☐ A *Bedol*
  ☐ B *Elleste-Solo*
  ☐ C *FemSeven*
  ☐ D *Premique*
  ☐ E *Premarin*

19 Which of the following is the most effective method of contraception?

  ☐ A condoms
  ☐ B copper coil
  ☐ C hormonal contraception
  ☐ D lubricating jelly
  ☐ E spermicides

Questions 20–21 concern the use of drugs in Mrs LB, a 31-year-old woman who is 35 weeks pregnant with her second child and presents at your pharmacy.

20 Mrs LB asks for some pain relief as she has had a painful back since last night. The counter assistant refers her to you as she is pregnant. Assuming she is not allergic or sensitive to anything, which of the following would be the safest analgesic product to sell to her?

  ☐ A aspirin tablets
  ☐ B caffeine based tablets
  ☐ C codeine based tablets
  ☐ D ibuprofen tablets
  ☐ E paracetamol tablets

21 One month later, Mrs LB presents again for some advice. She has recently given birth and is unsure as to whether she should be breast-feeding while on her regular prescribed medications. Which drug on her prescription may not be suitable for her during the first few weeks after birth?

    ☐ A   bendroflumethiazide
    ☐ B   enalapril
    ☐ C   insulin aspart
    ☐ D   labetalol
    ☐ E   paracetamol

Questions 22–25 concern the supply of medication from your community pharmacy for various patients who present with NHS prescriptions.

22 The local GP has prescribed sildenafil on an FP10 form for Mr KM, a diabetic patient who has erectile dysfunction. What endorsement is required on the prescription to authorise the dispensing of this drug?

    ☐ A   ACBS
    ☐ B   BB
    ☐ C   PC
    ☐ D   PNC
    ☐ E   SLS

23 Which of the following preparations is considered by the Joint Formulary Committee to be less suitable for prescribing?

    ☐ A   co-amoxiclav
    ☐ B   co-codamol
    ☐ C   co-cyprindiol
    ☐ D   co-dydramol
    ☐ E   co-phenotrope

24 Mr BW, a 52-year-old contractor who normally pays for his prescription, presents with an FP10 for the following items:

> Warfarin 1 mg tablets
> Warfarin 3 mg tablets
> Warfarin 5 mg tablets

How many NHS prescription charges should you levy?

> ☐ **A** 0
> ☐ **B** 1
> ☐ **C** 2
> ☐ **D** 3
> ☐ **E** 4

25 Miss SY, a 23-year-old dentist who normally pays for her prescription, presents with an FP10 for the following items:

> *Cilest* tablets
> Mefenamic acid tablets
> Tranexamic acid tablets

How many NHS prescription charges should you levy?

> ☐ **A** 0
> ☐ **B** 1
> ☐ **C** 2
> ☐ **D** 3
> ☐ **E** 4

26 You receive an urgent call from the hospital paediatric registrar regarding a child for whom he has just reviewed some medical results. The results show that the child has glucose-6-phosphate dehydrogenase deficiency. The registrar needs to prescribe an antibiotic for a urinary tract infection. Which of the following drugs carries a definite risk of haemolysis?

> ☐ **A** amoxicillin
> ☐ **B** cefalexin
> ☐ **C** co-amoxiclav
> ☐ **D** nitrofurantoin
> ☐ **E** trimethoprim

27 Mrs SM comes to your pharmacy for some advice. She has been told in a recent allergy test that she is allergic to sorbic acid, and that this has an 'E' number. Which one of the following is the correct E number for sorbic acid?

  ☐ A   E102
  ☐ B   E104
  ☐ C   E200
  ☐ D   E211
  ☐ E   E320

28 A patient on your ward who is being treated for schizophrenia is unresponsive to chlorpromazine (100 mg TDS) and is due to be switched to clozapine. The medical team asks for your advice as to an equivalent total daily dose of clozapine. Which one of the following is the total daily dose of clozapine equivalent to that of chlorpromazine?

  ☐ A   50 mg
  ☐ B   100 mg
  ☐ C   150 mg
  ☐ D   200 mg
  ☐ E   250 mg

29 Which one of the following conditions is not a caution for administering atenolol tablets to a patient?

  ☐ A   COPD
  ☐ B   diabetes
  ☐ C   myasthenia gravis
  ☐ D   pregnancy
  ☐ E   psoriasis

30 The pre-registration pharmacist at your local hospital comes across a patient newly started on amiodarone. As the ward pharmacist, he asks you to explain any monitoring required with this drug. Which of the following monitoring parameters is not required prior to initiating amiodarone?

  ☐ A   chest radiograph
  ☐ B   echocardiogram
  ☐ C   liver function tests
  ☐ D   serum potassium level
  ☐ E   thyroid function tests

31 Mr KF presents to hospital with an inflammatory condition. His drug history shows that he currently takes prednisolone tablets (10 mg daily). The doctor on the ward would like to change the drug to hydrocortisone, which has a greater anti-inflammatory action. What dose of hydrocortisone tablets should the doctor prescribe?

    ☐ A   5 mg
    ☐ B   10 mg
    ☐ C   20 mg
    ☐ D   40 mg
    ☐ E   60 mg

32 Mrs SC visits her GP as she has a persistent dry cough that is keeping her awake at night. Her GP decides to change her regular medication, ramipril, as he attributes the cough to this drug. Which one of the following would be the most suitable alternative?

    ☐ A   amlodipine
    ☐ B   atenolol
    ☐ C   chlortalidone
    ☐ D   doxazosin
    ☐ E   irbesartan

33 Your local GP phones you for advice. He wants to prescribe a 'mildly potent' topical corticosteroid.
Which one do you advise?

    ☐ A   *Betnovate* RD cream
    ☐ B   *Diprosone cream*
    ☐ C   *Eumovate* cream
    ☐ D   *Nerisone Forte* cream
    ☐ E   *Synalar* 1 in 10 cream

34 You are asked to supply *Betnovate* cream for Mr GS, a patient on your ward, who is suffering from an eczema flare-up. Mr GS will need to apply the cream twice daily for two weeks to his legs and trunk.
How many 100 g tubes of this product should you supply to cover the two-week period?

    ☐ A   1
    ☐ B   2
    ☐ C   3
    ☐ D   4
    ☐ E   5

35 Mrs JT has recently been prescribed hormone replacement therapy (HRT). You counsel her on her new medication and mention possible side-effects that may occur and situations when she should stop her HRT immediately. Which of the following is not a reason for Mrs JT to stop her HRT treatment?

- [ ] A breast tenderness
- [ ] B calf pain
- [ ] C abdominal pain
- [ ] D chest pain
- [ ] E prolonged headache

36 The nutrition team prescribe *Kabiven* (1026 mL) for a patient who requires parenteral feeding. Approximately how many millimoles of magnesium ions per litre does this bag contain?

- [ ] A 2.5
- [ ] B 2.8
- [ ] C 4.0
- [ ] D 4.5
- [ ] E 5.0

37 A cardiac house officer asks for you to counsel Mr KB, a patient he has newly initiated on amiodarone for Wolff-Parkinson-White syndrome. Which of the following is unsuitable advice for you to provide Mr KB?

- [ ] A Mr KB needs to take amiodarone three times a day for the first week.
- [ ] B Mr KB needs to protect his skin using sunscreen as amiodarone is phototoxic.
- [ ] C Mr KB will need thyroid function monitoring as amiodarone can affect this.
- [ ] D Mr KB can continue taking amiodarone if he suffers shortness of breath.
- [ ] E Mr KB must inform a doctor if he gets dazzled by headlights when driving at night.

38 The pain sister asks for your advice regarding Mrs DW who has been receiving morphine sulfate 120 mg twice daily. She would like to change her to diamorphine subcutaneous infusion every 24 hours. What should the initial daily dose of diamorphine via a subcutaneous infusion be?

    □ A   20 mg
    □ B   40 mg
    □ C   60 mg
    □ D   80 mg
    □ E   120 mg

39 Mrs SG comes to your pharmacy complaining that she has been constipated for three days due to her recently starting dried ferrous sulfate 200 mg tablets (at a dose of 200 mg TDS). She insists that she would like an alternative iron salt. Which of the following preparations at the said dose and frequency will provide a similar amount of ferrous iron as her current tablets?

    □ A   *Fersaday tablets*   1 tablet BD
    □ B   *Fersamal syrup*   10 mL BD
    □ C   *Galfer capsules*   1 capsule BD
    □ D   *Ironorm drops*   0.6 mL OD
    □ E   *Sytron elixir*   10 mL BD

40 You are on call and one of the ward sisters pages you to find out which diluent to use with *Ambisome* and what the recommended method of infusion is. Which of the following tabulated options is correct?

		Diluent	Method of infusion
□	A	Compound Sodium Lactate Solution	Intermittent
□	B	Glucose 5%	Continuous
□	C	Glucose 5%	Intermittent
□	D	Sodium Chloride 0.9%	Continuous
□	E	Sodium Chloride 0.9%	Intermittent

41 Mrs AG is taking clomipramine for depression. She is due to be swapped to phenelzine. How long should Mrs AG's doctor wait before asking her to start her phenelzine?

    □ A   1 week
    □ B   2 weeks
    □ C   3 weeks
    □ D   4 weeks
    □ E   5 weeks

42 A patient on your ward has just been started on numerous medications. You check for cautions and interactions on his prescription chart. Which of the following combinations from his prescription chart does not have a potential caution or interaction when used concomitantly?

    □ A   alendronic acid and *Adcal D3*
    □ B   amphotericin and prednisolone
    □ C   ciprofloxacin and ferrous sulfate
    □ D   ondansetron and voriconazole
    □ E   prednisolone and *Zineryt*

43 Mr AS has returned some buprenorphine 2.5 mcg patches to your pharmacy as he no longer uses them. Assuming you have a witness, which of the following options is the most appropriate manner in which to destroy the patches?

    □ A   Cut the patches into small parts and throw in a special waste bin.
    □ B   Place the patches into a small amount of soapy water.
    □ C   Place the patches into a denaturing kit.
    □ D   Throw the patches into the 'sharps' bin.
    □ E   Remove the backing paper and fold patches upon themselves.

44 Mr FZ is a 45-year-old with an average blood pressure of 180/95 mmHg and a serum total cholesterol to HDL cholesterol ratio of 8. He has no past medical history and does not smoke. What is the percentage cardiovascular risk prediction for Mr FZ over the next 10 years?

    □ A   <15%
    □ B   >15%
    □ C   10–20%
    □ D   >20%
    □ E   >30%

45 A prescription is brought to your pharmacy for *Zomig*. You wish to check the approved name for this drug so that you can check the dose and potential interactions with any of the customer's current medication. What is the approved name of the medicine on the prescription?

    ☐ A   almotriptan
    ☐ B   naratriptan
    ☐ C   pizotifen
    ☐ D   sumatriptan
    ☐ E   zolmitriptan

46 A doctor wishes to prescribe some *Copegus* capsules for Mr FP who is 32 years old and weighs 66 kg. Mr FP has a history of HIV, and has just been diagnosed with chronic hepatitis C. The doctor asks you to suggest a dose for Mr FP who has 'normal' renal function. What dose regimen is most suitable?

    ☐ A   400 mg twice daily
    ☐ B   400 mg in the morning and 600 mg in the evening
    ☐ C   600 mg twice daily
    ☐ D   600 mg in the morning and 400 mg in the evening
    ☐ E   200 mg in the morning and 400 mg in the evening

47 Assuming no cautions or contraindications apply, which of the following products is not available for counter-prescribing for the listed indication and patient?

    ☐ A   Hydrocortisone 1% cream for eczema in a 12-year-old child.
    ☐ B   Clobetasone butyrate 0.05% cream for seborrhoeic dermatitis in a 12-year-old child.
    ☐ C   Diclofenac 2.32% gel for musculoskeletal pain in an 18-year-old football player.
    ☐ D   Ibuprofen 5% gel for rheumatic pain in a 45-year-old-builder.
    ☐ E   Miconazole 2% cream in a 33-year-old man with a fungal nail infection.

48 Child SC who is 6 years old and weighs 15 kg requires intramuscular adrenaline (epinephrine) due to an anaphylactic reaction he has had to some cashew nuts. Which of the following doses of intramuscular adrenaline (epinephrine) would be most suitable for him?

    □ A   50 mcg
    □ B   100 mcg
    □ C   150 mcg
    □ D   300 mcg
    □ E   500 mcg

49 Mr SG comes to your pharmacy asking you to recommend something for his sore throat and fever. You check his patient medication record (PMR) and decide to immediately refer him to the nearest hospital emergency department. Which of the following drugs from his PMR gave you cause for concern?

    □ A   aspirin
    □ B   carbimazole
    □ C   enalapril
    □ D   hydrocortisone ointment
    □ E   pravastatin

50 Which of the following chemotherapy drugs may be administered intrathecally?

    □ A   cytarabine
    □ B   doxorubicin
    □ C   vincristine
    □ D   vindesine
    □ E   vinorelbine

MULTIPLE COMPLETION QUESTIONS

Oksana Pyzik

Each of the questions or incomplete statements in this section is followed by three responses. For each question, ONE or MORE of the responses is/are correct. Decide which of the responses is/are correct, then choose:

A   if **1, 2,** and **3** are correct
B   if **1** and **2** only are correct
C   if **2** and **3** only are correct
D   if **1** only is correct
E   if **3** only is correct

Summary				
A	B	C	D	E
1, 2, 3	1, 2 only	2, 3 only	1 only	3 only

1   Which of the following antiviral agents are active against cytomegalovirus (CMV)?

    ☐ **1**   aciclovir
    ☐ **2**   ganciclovir
    ☐ **3**   foscarnet

2   You are on call and the sister on one of the wards asks for your advice. She has different ferric complexes on the ward, but is not sure which one(s) she can give parenterally.
    What advice do you give about the following?

    ☐ **1**   iron isomaltoside 1000
    ☐ **2**   ferumoxytol
    ☐ **3**   iron sucrose

3   Mr Wilson is a cancer patient who is experiencing severe nausea and vomiting as a result of the chemotherapy treatment. Which of the following drugs from his PMR are classified as highly emetogenic?

    ☐ **1**   fluorouracil
    ☐ **2**   dacarbazine
    ☐ **3**   cisplatin

4   Mr Nederpel is admitted to hospital for a severe infection and is flagged as a high-risk patient. He has a history of seizures and has moderately impaired drug elimination. Upon reviewing his drug chart, which of the following medicines will require careful monitoring for drug-related seizures?

    ☐ 1   metronidazole
    ☐ 2   benzylpenicillin
    ☐ 3   amphotericin B

5   A 31-year-old woman comes to the pharmacy asking for *Levonelle*. She had unprotected sex 52 hours ago and is on no other medicines but has acute porphyria. You decide not to supply it because:

    ☐ 1   emergency contraception is not available without a prescription
    ☐ 2   emergency contraception is not effective within 52 hours of unprotected sex
    ☐ 3   emergency contraception is contraindicated for this patient.

6   Difficulties in adherence to drug treatment occur regardless of age, but for children, which of the following may be most relevant?

    ☐ 1   Difficulty in taking the medicine, such as the inability to swallow the medicine.
    ☐ 2   Unattractive formulation. such as unpleasant taste.
    ☐ 3   Carer's or child's perception of the risk and severity of side-effects may differ from that of the prescriber.

7   Which of the following statements regarding wholesale dealing is correct?

    ☐ 1   Persons trading in medicines should apply Good Distribution Practice.
    ☐ 2   According to the MHRA, as of August 2012, a pharmacist engaging in commercial trading in medicines does not need to hold a Wholesale Dealer's Licence.
    ☐ 3   All healthcare professionals can receive medications by wholesale.

8   With regard to veterinary medicines, which of the following details must appear on your dispensing label when you supply a product for use 'under the cascade'?

    ☐ 1   Identification of the animal.
    ☐ 2   Withdrawal period (if there is one).
    ☐ 3   The words for 'animal treatment only'.

9   The sister on your ward asks for some advice for one of the terminally ill patients. A syringe driver needs to be set up with diamorphine subcutaneously. The doctors have prescribed some other drugs, which are also to be added to the syringe driver.
   Which of the following drug(s) is/are compatible with diamorphine?

   ☐ 1   haloperidol
   ☐ 2   midazolam
   ☐ 3   hyoscine butylbromide

10 Which of the following medicines can cause kidney stones?

   ☐ 1   topiramate
   ☐ 2   phenytoin
   ☐ 3   vigabatrin

11 Scott is a 38-year-old male who is being treated at the hospital for severe renal impairment, and his electrolyte levels are being closely monitored. Which of the following electrolytes would you expect to increase?

   ☐ 1   phosphate
   ☐ 2   potassium
   ☐ 3   calcium

12 You have a woman on your gynaecology ward for whom the doctor wants to prescribe an HRT preparation. The patient had a hysterectomy about one year ago.
   Which preparation(s) would be suited to her?

   ☐ 1   *Elleste-Solo* tablets
   ☐ 2   Progynova
   ☐ 3   Premique

13 A concerned lady comes to your pharmacy and gives you a list of drugs that her GP has just prescribed for her. She forgot to tell her GP that she is still breastfeeding her baby.
   Which drugs from her prescription should she avoid?

   ☐ 1   gliclazide
   ☐ 2   tetracycline
   ☐ 3   tolterodine

14 Mr Franco is a patient on your ward with *severe* liver failure. Which of the following is not a symptom of liver failure?

☐ 1 finger clubbing
☐ 2 ascites
☐ 3 pulmonary oedema

15 A child of two months requires which of the following vaccines?

☐ 1 diphtheria
☐ 2 pneumococcal polysaccharide conjugate vaccine
☐ 3 meningococcal group C conjugate vaccine

16 Which of the following drugs may cause blood disorders?

☐ 1 tranylcypromine
☐ 2 desferrioxamine mesilate
☐ 3 trimethoprim

17 Hypothermia may develop in patients of any age who have been deeply unconscious for some hours, particularly following overdose with which of the following medicines?

☐ 1 barbiturates
☐ 2 phenothiazines
☐ 3 diphenhydramine

18 Which of the following statements is/are correct regarding Patient Group Directives (PGDs)?

☐ 1 Are written directions, allowing the supply and/or administration of a specified medicine (or medicines) by named healthcare professionals to a well-defined group of patients requiring treatment for a specific condition.
☐ 2 Allow pharmacists to supply diamorphine or morphine for the immediate necessary treatment of sick or injured persons, in accordance with the terms set out in a PGD.
☐ 3 Should be drawn-up by a multidisciplinary group involving a doctor, a pharmacist, and a representative of any professional group expected to supply medicines under the PGD.

19 Long-term use of opioids can cause which of the following?

☐ 1   hyperalgesia
☐ 2   hypogonadism
☐ 3   adrenal insufficiency

20 Which of the following atypical antipsychotics is/are most likely to cause weight gain as a side-effect?

☐ 1   aripiprazole
☐ 2   olanzapine
☐ 3   clozapine

21 AW suffers from heart failure and is taking digoxin. Which of the following electrolyte imbalances predispose AW to digitalis toxicity?

☐ 1   hypermagnesaemia
☐ 2   hyperkalaemia
☐ 3   hypercalcaemia

22 A GP telephones asking for some advice. He wants to withdraw prednisolone tablets from one of his patients. The Committee on Safety of Medicines (CSM) advises that gradual withdrawal should be considered in those whose disease is unlikely to relapse and

☐ 1   in patients who have taken a short course within one year of stopping long-term therapy
☐ 2   in patients who have received more than 40 mg daily of prednisolone
☐ 3   in patients who have received more than three weeks' treatment.

23 Mrs Van Loon is a patient on your ward with severe rheumatoid arthritis and has been taking leflunomide for the past year. However, her doctor wants to change her to another disease modifying antirheumatic drug. Which of the following washout procedures would be appropriate?

☐ 1   Stop current treatment and start new treatment after 7 days.
☐ 2   Stop current treatment and give colestyramine 8 g TDS for 11 days.
☐ 3   Stop current treatment and give charcoal 50 g q.d.s. for 11 days.

24 You are working with the Macmillan palliative care team in your hospital. One of the doctors asks you about the licensing of dexrazoxane. Which of the following is/are correct?

☐ 1 Prevention of chronic cumulative cardiotoxicity caused by doxorubicin in patients with advanced breast cancer who have received a prior cumulative dose of $300\,mg/m^2$.

☐ 2 Prevention of chronic cumulative cardiotoxicity caused by epirubicin in metastatic breast cancer who have received a prior cumulative dose of $540\,mg/m^2$.

☐ 3 Treatment of anthracycline extravasation.

25 Some Latin abbreviations are used in prescribing. Which of the following abbreviations match with the correct translation?

☐ 1 p.c. = post cibum
☐ 2 q.q.h. = quarta quaque hora
☐ 3 o.m. = omni mane

26 A doctor wants to prescribe strontium ranelate for one of his patients and asks you if it is safe for this patient. From the following, in which group(s) of patients is this drug contraindicated?

☐ 1 Patients who are temporarily immobile or for prolonged periods.
☐ 2 Patients with uncontrolled hypertension.
☐ 3 Patients with a current or previous venous thromboembolic event.

27 KM is currently on hormone replacement therapy. Which of the following is/are contraindications?

☐ 1 epilepsy
☐ 2 liver disease
☐ 3 deep vein thrombosis

28 A pregnant woman exposed to teratogenic drugs could cause fetal abnormalities during which of the following times?

☐ 1 fetal period
☐ 2 weeks 3–8 of gestation
☐ 3 first two weeks of gestation

29 Which of the following is true regarding gentamicin?

  □ 1 There is an increased risk of nephrotoxicity when given concomitantly with ciclosporin.
  □ 2 There is an increased risk of ototoxicity when given concomitantly with furosemide.
  □ 3 There is an increased risk of hypocalcaemia when given concomitantly with alendronic acid.

30 You are working for the medicines information department in your hospital. The obstetrics senior house officer telephones to ask your advice. He has a pregnant patient who is diabetic and would like to know the most appropriate antidiabetic medication for her.
   Which of the following would be appropriate for her?

  □ 1 insulin
  □ 2 metformin
  □ 3 gliclazide

31 Identify the correct statements regarding oxytocin:

  □ 1 Uterotonic effect of oxytocin is potentiated by prostaglandins.
  □ 2 General anaesthetics reduce the oxytocic effect.
  □ 3 There is an enhanced risk of arrhythmias when oxytocin is given with volatile liquid general anaesthetics.

32 Self-monitoring of blood-glucose concentration is appropriate for patients with type 2 diabetes:

  □ 1 who are treated with sulfonylureas
  □ 2 who are treated with insulin
  □ 3 to monitor changes in blood-glucose concentration resulting from changes in lifestyle or medication, and during intercurrent illness.

33 Drugs associated with prolonged QT intervals include:

  □ 1 clarithromycin
  □ 2 lithium
  □ 3 enalapril

34 CD is one of your regular customers. She brings in a prescription for *Fosamax*. She has never had these tablets before. You counsel her on the new tablets. Which points are specific to this drug?

☐ **1**   Swallow whole.
☐ **2**   Do not take the tablets at bedtime or before rising.
☐ **3**   These tablets may cause drowsiness.

35 A senior registrar in obstetrics wants to prescribe dinoprostone to induce labour in one of his patients. He contacts you to check whether this drug is contraindicated in his patient.
In which of the following circumstances is this drug contraindicated?

☐ **1**   Patients with a history of caesarean section.
☐ **2**   Patients with renal disease.
☐ **3**   Patients who have had unexplained bleeding during pregnancy.

36 Prolonged use can exaggerate some of the normal physiological actions of corticosteroids leading to mineralocorticoid side-effects such as:

☐ **1**   hypotension
☐ **2**   sodium and water retention
☐ **3**   potassium and calcium loss

37 Which of the following is/are true regarding glucose-6-phosphate dehydrogenase deficiency?

☐ **1**   Moth balls may cause haemolysis in these individuals.
☐ **2**   The risk and severity of haemolysis due to taking a drug is almost always dose related.
☐ **3**   The deficiency is prevalent in individuals originating from southern Europe.

38 Which of the following cytotoxic drugs cause bone marrow depression?

☐ **1**   bleomycin
☐ **2**   vincristine
☐ **3**   cyclophosphamide

39 One of your patients on the ward has recently developed severe hyponatraemia. You check the drug chart to see if any of his drugs may be the cause.
Which of the following drug(s) may cause hyponatraemia?

☐ **1**   propranolol
☐ **2**   bumetanide
☐ **3**   fluoxetine

40 A patient on your ward has severe renal impairment.
Which drugs should be avoided?

☐ 1 buspirone
☐ 2 ropinirole
☐ 3 tinzaparin

41 Which person(s) from the following list is/are permitted to supply or administer under patient group directions?

☐ 1 pharmacists
☐ 2 dentists
☐ 3 doctors

42 In neonates, gonococcal eye infections may be treated with which of the following courses of licensed treatment?

☐ 1 Single dose of parenteral cefotaxime.
☐ 2 Single dose of parenteral ceftriaxone.
☐ 3 Gentamicin 1.5% eye drops.

43 Which of the following medicines may exacerbate gout?

☐ 1 bendroflumethiazide
☐ 2 furosemide
☐ 3 aspirin

44 The pertussis vaccine should not be withheld from children with a history of preceding dose of:

☐ 1 fever, irrespective of severity
☐ 2 persistent crying or screaming for more than 3 hours
☐ 3 severe local reaction, irrespective of extent.

45 Mrs Tso's GP has prescribed *Trimovate* cream for her 6-month-old baby's eczema. She is very concerned about using a topical corticosteroid and asks you about the side-effects.
Which of the below is/are a side-effect of the cream?

☐ 1 irreversible striae
☐ 2 thinning of the skin
☐ 3 mild reversible depigmentation

46 In children, thyroid hormones are used to treat which of the following conditions?

- ☐ 1 juvenille myxoedema
- ☐ 2 diffuse non-toxic goitre
- ☐ 3 lymphadenoid goitre

47 Which person(s) is/are authorised to supervise the destruction of controlled drugs?

- ☐ 1 Home Office inspector
- ☐ 2 Royal Pharmaceutical Society inspector
- ☐ 3 Registered General Medical Council doctor

48 Which of the following statements is/are true with regard to the appropriate protocol for the withdrawal of prescribed long-term benzodiazepines?

- ☐ 1 Benzodiazepine withdrawal symptoms for long-term users usually resolve within 6–18 months of the last dose.
- ☐ 2 Benzodiazepine dose reduction rate should be flexible.
- ☐ 3 Add antidepressants to therapy if withdrawal symptoms persist.

49 A lady comes into your pharmacy for some advice. She normally takes *Microgynon* every day at 9 p.m. She is in the middle of her cycle and forgot to take her pill last night and is not sure what she should do. Given that it is 11 a.m. when she comes to see you, what advice do you give?

- ☐ 1 Take a pill straight away, then take the next one at her normal time.
- ☐ 2 She must use condoms for the next seven days or abstain from sex.
- ☐ 3 Miss out the seven inactive pills for the following month.

50 Which of the following cardiac enzymes and biomarkers exhibit the highest specificity and sensitivity for the diagnosis of acute myocardial infarction?

- ☐ 1 C-reactive protein (CRP)
- ☐ 2 creatine kinase (CK-MB)
- ☐ 3 troponins T and I

CLASSIFICATION QUESTIONS

Alistair Murray

In this section, for each numbered question, select the one lettered option that most closely corresponds to the answer. Within each group of questions each lettered option may be used once, more than once, or not at all.

Questions 1–4 concern the following names for E numbers:

A ponceau 4R
B butylated hydroxyanisole
C glycerol
D sorbic acid
E lecithins

What are the names for the following E numbers?

1 E200
2 E320
3 E124
4 E322

Questions 5–8 concern the following drugs:

A carbamazepine
B lithium
C verapamil
D theophylline
E azathioprine

Which of the above drugs are considered to have a potentially serious interaction with the following:

5 allopurinol
6 bendroflumethiazide
7 bisoprolol
8 chlorpromazine

Questions 9–12 concern the following drugs:

A   apraclonidine
B   codeine phosphate
C   epoetin alfa
D   folic acid
E   buprenorphine

On your ward you have seen some drugs that you do not recognise. You want to find out what their indications are.
Match the drugs with the indications below:

9   control of intraocular pressure
10 anaemia associated with chronic renal failure
11 moderate to severe pain
12 prevention of spina bifida in pregnancy

Questions 13–16 concern the following drugs:

A   oxytetracycline 250 mg tablets
B   nitrofurantoin 100 mg capsules
C   clarithromycin 250 mg tablets
D   erythromycin 250 mg tablets
E   doxycycline 100 mg capsules

Match the correct drugs with the cautionary labels:

13 Do not take indigestion remedies 2 hours before or after you take this medicine.
14 Do not take milk, indigestion remedies, or medicines containing iron or zinc, 2 hours before or after you take this medicine.
15 This medicine may colour your urine. This is harmless.
16 Do not take indigestion remedies, or medicines containing iron or zinc, 2 hours before or after you take this medicine.

Questions 17–20 concern the following drugs:

A   ciprofloxacin
B   metformin
C   salbutamol
D   glucagon
E   gliclazide

Which of the above drugs:

17 is used for the inhibition of premature labour?
18 is used to treat hypoglycaemia?
19 may cause haemolytic anaemia in patients with a G6PD deficiency?
20 is used as a first-line antidiabetic treatment in overweight patients?

Questions 21–24 concern the following drugs:

    A   adrenaline/epinephrine
    B   ispaghula
    C   simvastatin
    D   amitriptyline
    E   octreotide

Which of the above drugs:

21 is used in the treatment of anaphylaxis?
22 is contraindicated in patients who have had a recent myocardial infarction?
23 can cause dry eyes as a side-effect?
24 is used to treat acromegaly?

For questions 25–28, choose from the following list:

    A   Not allowed
    B   One
    C   Two
    D   Three
    E   None

Mrs F is a paient at your pharmacy and she normally pays for her prescriptions. She is being treated for trigeminal neuralgia.
How many NHS charges would she have to pay for the following items?

25 *Femodette* tablets × 42 (2 OP)
26 *Scholl* thigh length stockings, class III × 1 pair
27 paracetamol 500 mg tablets × 100
28 carbamazepine 200 mg tablets × 3 OP

Questions 29–32 concern the following drugs:

A   temazepam 10 mg tablets
B   *MST Continus* 10 mg tablets
C   diazepam 10 mg/2 mL injection
D   dexamfetamine 5 mg tablets
E   cannabis

Which of the above drugs:

29 may be given as an emergency supply?
30 is a schedule 1 controlled drug?
31 is used in the treatment of epilepsy?
32 is used in the treatment of narcolepsy?

Questions 33–36 concern the following drugs:

A   cilostazol
B   tizanidine
C   sodium nitroprusside
D   pregabalin
E   adrenaline

Which of the above drugs:

33 can be used for the treatment of neuropathic pain?
34 can be used in the treatment of peripheral vascular disease?
35 can be used for the treatment of hypertensive crisis?
36 can be used for the short-term relief of muscle spasm?

Questions 37–40 concern the following side-effects:

A   folate deficiency
B   disturbance in colour vision
C   constipation
D   hyperthyroidism
E   heart toxicity

Match the side-effects caused by the drugs below:

37 potassium chloride
38 methotrexate
39 amiodarone
40 ethambutol

Questions 41–45 concern the following side-effects:

A hyperkalaemia
B hypercalcaemia
C hyponatraemia
D hypokalaemia
E hypernatraemia

Match the side-effects caused by the drugs below:

41 *Desmotabs* 200 mcg tablets
42 *Priadel* 200 mg m/r tablets
43 spironolactone 50 mg tablets
44 *Dovonex* ointment
45 *Bricanyl* respules 5 mg/2 mL

For questions 46–50, choose from the following list:

A Medix Lifecare Nebuliser System
B Pocket Chamber
C *Benadryl* 8 mg capsules
D Mini-Wright peak flow meter
E *Sudafed* tablets

Which of the above:

46 has been deemed less suitable for prescribing by the Joint Formulary Committee?
47 cannot be prescribed on the NHS?
48 is used for monitoring respiratory symptoms?
49 is contraindicated in patients with hypersensitivity to tripolidine?
50 is used to improve inhaler technique?

STATEMENT QUESTIONS

Ryan Hamilton

> The questions in this section consist of a statement in the top row followed by a second statement beneath.
>
> You need to:
>
> decide whether the *first statement* is true or false
>
> decide whether the *second statement* is true or false
>
> Then choose:
>
> A　if both statements are true and the second statement is *a correct explanation* of the first statement
>
> B　if both statements are true but the second statement is *not a correct explanation* of the first statement
>
> C　if the first statement is true but the second statement is false
>
> D　if the first statement is false but the second statement is true
>
> E　if both statements are false

1　**First statement**

Gastrocote tablets should be used with caution in diabetic patients with dyspepsia

Second statement

Gastrocote tablets have a high sugar content

2　**First statement**

All H_2-receptor antagonists heal gastric and duodenal ulcers

Second statement

H_2-antagonists reduce gastric acid secretion as a result of H_2-receptor blockade

3　**First statement**

Ivabradine is a drug that lowers heart rate

Second statement

Ivabradine acts on the bundle of His to slow electrical impulses

4 **First statement**

Atypical antipsychotics should be considered when choosing first-line pharmacological treatment of newly diagnosed schizophrenia

Second statement

Olanzapine is associated with an increased risk of stroke in elderly patients with dementia

5 **First statement**

Nausea in the first trimester of pregnancy is usually mild

Second statement

Metoclopramide should be given as first-line treatment for mild nausea in pregnancy

6 **First statement**

Pethidine should be avoided in patients with sickle-cell disease

Second statement

Pethidine can precipitate gout

7 **First statement**

Potassium should be monitored in patients prescribed ciclosporin therapy

Second statement

Ciclosporin may cause hyperkalaemia

8 **First statement**

Peptac liquid is suitable for patients with dyspepsia who also have hypertension

Second statement

Peptac liquid is a low-sodium preparation

9 **First statement**

Patients taking dopaminergic drugs should exercise caution when driving

Second statement

Dopaminergic drugs can cause a sudden onset of sleep at any time during the day or night

10 **First statement**

Mifepristone is used for the induction of labour in normal pregnancy

Second statement

Mifepristone sensitises the myometrium to prostaglandin-induced contractions and ripens the cervix

11 **First statement**

Diabetic ketoacidosis may induce hyponatraemia

Second statement

Sodium chloride in isotonic solution is indicated for hyponatraemia induced by diabetic ketoacidosis

12 **First statement**

Vitamin C deficiency causes rickets

Second statement

Vitamin C is a fat-soluble vitamin

13 **First statement**

Penicillamine is used in the treatment of Wilson's disease

Second statement

Penicillamine aids the elimination of magnesium ions

14 **First statement**

Artificial saliva can be prescribed for patients with a dry mouth

Second statement

Tricyclic antidepressants can cause dry mouth

15 **First statement**

Patients taking methotrexate should report signs of infection, especially sore throat

Second statement

Methotrexate therapy may induce agranulocystosis

16 **First statement**

Darunavir interacts with St John's wort

Second statement

St John's wort reduces the serum concentration of darunavir

17 **First statement**

Ganciclovir can be given safely in pregnancy

Second statement

Ganciclovir does not cross the placenta

18 **First statement**

Eprex is given by subcutaneous injection to treat anaemia caused by renal failure

Second statement

Eprex mimics the action of endogenous erythropoietin

19 **First statement**

Aqueous cream should not be used to treat eczema in children

Second statement

Aqueous cream contains sodium lauryl sulfate

20 **First statement**

Hydrocortisone 0.5% cream for use on the face should be prescribed in quantities of 15 g

Second statement

Hydrocortisone is a strong corticosteroid

Question 21 concerns the following scenario:

Mrs L weighs 45 kg and requires IV paracetamol for control of postoperative pain.

21 **First statement**

To avoid liver damage, Mrs L should receive no more than three doses of paracetamol in any 24-hour period.

Second statement

The paracetamol dose should be calculated at 15 mg/kg

22 **First statement**

Patients taking verapamil should not be prescribed simvastatin at a dose greater than 10 mg daily

Second statement

Simvastatin can increase the serum concentration of verapamil

23 **First statement**

Vincristine should not be administered intrathecally

Second statement

Peripheral and autonomic neuropathy may become intolerable for patients receiving vincristine.

24 **First statement**

Cephalosporins should be used with caution in patients with a history of penicillin allergy

Second statement

Cephalosporins belong to the penicillin-class of antibacterial drugs.

Questions 25 and 26 concern the following scenario:

Mrs H is an asymptomatic HIV positive patient whose immunity is not yet significantly impaired. Her GP asks you some questions about vaccinations.

25 **First statement**

Mrs H should not receive the *Zostavax* vaccine

Second statement

Zostavax contains a live attenuated strain of the varicella-zoster virus

26 **First statement**

Mrs H should receive the seasonal flu vaccine every year

Second statement

The nasal route would be the most suitable way to vaccinate Mrs H against flu

27 **First statement**

Calcium alginate dressings are suitable for most exudating wounds

Second statement

Calcium alginate dressings promote homeostasis within the wound-bed

Question 28 concerns the following scenario:

Mr S comes into your community pharmacy to talk to you about stopping smoking. He currently smokes 20 cigarettes a day and wants to try an electronic cigarette.

28 **First statement**

You should discuss all treatment options with Mr S, not just the role of electronic cigarettes

Second statement

There is no long-term safety data to support the use of electronic cigarettes

Question 29 concerns the following scenario:

Mrs P phones your community pharmacy because her three-year-old daughter has accessed their bottle of paracetamol 120 mg/5 mL oral suspension. On further questioning, you believe she may have taken about 20 mL of the suspension.

29 **First statement**

You should reassure Mrs P that there is no immediate risk of overdose to her daughter and no further action is needed.

Second statement

Acute overdose of 75 mg/kg, or more, taken within one hour will rarely lead to liver damage

Questions 30–32 concern the following scenario:

A four-year-old patient, Charlie, has been newly diagnosed with asthma and prescribed a *Ventolin Evohaler.*

30 **First statement**

Charlie should also be prescribed a spacer

Second statement

The spacer should be rinsed with water after every use

31 **First statement**

In the event of an asthma attack, Charlie should inhale up to ten doses of *Ventolin*, performing tidal breathing between each actuation

Second statement

Tidal breathing with a spacer is as good as a nebuliser at treating mild and moderate acute exacerbations of asthma

32 **First statement**

Charlie should receive the seasonal flu vaccination every year

Second statement

Fluenz provides more protection than the intramuscular injection

Questions 33 and 34 concern the following scenario:

Mrs W is taking warfarin 4 mg daily for atrial fibrillation. At her recent anticoagulation clinic her INR was found to be 5.0. She is not taking any other medicines or made any lifestyle changes that could impact on the warfarin.

33 **First statement**

Mrs W should be advised to omit the next dose of warfarin

Second statement

The maintenance dose of warfarin will need to be reduced

34 **First statement**

An INR between 2.0 and 3.0 would be acceptable for Mrs W

Second statement

The target INR for Mrs W is 2.5

Question 35 concerns the following scenario:

A police officer has a court order requesting access to one of your patient's records.

35 **First statement**

You must disclose all the information you hold for this patient

Second statement

A court of law has automatic right to access all patient information

36 **First statement**

Clinical audits should be used to determine the performance of staff

Second statement

Clinical audits determine whether explicit standards and best practice are being met

37 **First statement**

Improvements should be proposed and implemented after each clinical audit

Second statement

A re-audit should be performed to determine whether the suggested improvements have been successful

38 **First statement**

Your CPD entries must meet all the assessable criteria for good recording practice as set by the GPhC

Second statement

Submitting CPD of insufficient quality can result in your removal from the register

39 **First statement**

Pharmacists should ensure patients do not stop taking their prescribed medicines if they are going to use homeopathy

Second statement

There is no scientific or clinical evidence to support the use of homeopathy

Question 40 concerns the following scenario:

George, an 11-year-old boy, comes into your community pharmacy to collect his regular asthma medicines.

40 **First statement**

You cannot supply the medicines to George because he is too young

Second statement

You need to be sure that George is capable and competent to understand the information he needs to use his medicines

41 **First statement**

Abidec should not be used to prevent vitamin deficiency in children who are allergic to nuts

Second statement

Abidec contains arachis oil

42 **First statement**

Sumatriptan can be supplied over the counter by a pharmacist for the treatment of migraine

Second statement

Sumatriptan can only be supplied to patients that have an established pattern of migraine

43 **First statement**

Insulin doses may need to be reduced in patients with renal impairment

Second statement

The compensatory response to hypoglycaemia is impaired in renal impairment

44 **First statement**

Sildenafil can be used to treat pulmonary hypertension in children

Second statement

Sildenafil inhibits the effects of nitric oxide, resulting in vasodilation

Question 45 concerns the following scenario:

A woman comes into your pharmacy on a Saturday morning requesting emergency hormonal contraception (EHC) without a prescription, following unprotected intercourse the night before.

45 **First statement**

You are able to decline to supply EHC if it contradicts your religious or moral beliefs

Second statement

You must refer the patient to their GP

Question 46 concerns the following scenario:

You are presented with an NHS dental prescription for erythromycin capsules.

46 **First statement**

You should ask the dentist to prescribe clindamycin capsules instead

Second statement

Erythromycin capsules are not listed in the Dental Practitioners' Formulary

Question 47 concerns the following scenario:

Mrs V presents a prescription to you for captopril oral liquid, 12.5 mg twice daily. You note that the prescription is for her 13-year-old son, Nitesh.

47 **First statement**

You should extemporaneously prepare this medicine in your pharmacy using captopril tablets

Second statement

There is no licensed liquid formulation of captopril

48 **First statement**

Patients taking phenytoin should receive the same brand and formulation each time it is dispensed

Second statement

Switching between formulations can result in loss of seizure control or increased incidence of adverse effects

49 **First statement**

Continuous subcutaneous infusions can be useful in palliative care for managing the symptoms of advanced cancer

Second statement

Diamorphine and hyoscine hydrobromide can be mixed and delivered in the same syringe

Question 50 concerns the following scenario:

> Mrs M has moderate (stage 3) renal impairment and has been admitted to your ward with a suspected urinary tract infection.

50 **First statement**

Mrs M should not be treated with nitrofurantoin

Second statement

Adequate urine concentrations of nitrofurantoin may not be achieved in this patient

Closed book questions

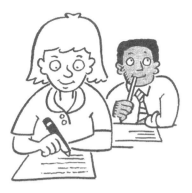

SIMPLE COMPLETION QUESTIONS

Ryan Hamilton

Each of the questions or statements in this section is followed by five suggested answers. Select the best answer in each situation.

Questions 1 and 2 concern the following scenario:

Mrs M has been admitted to your medical admissions unit with confusion and also suffers from rheumatoid arthritis for which she is prescribed methotrexate 10 mg once weekly, folic acid 5mg once weekly, and paracetamol 1 g four times a day. She has no known drug allergies.

1   The medical team diagnose Mrs M with a lower urinary tract infection and ask for your advice on the choice of treatment. Which of the following antibacterial agents would be the least appropriate to prescribe?

☐ A   amoxicillin
☐ B   cefalexin
☐ C   co-amoxiclav
☐ D   doxycycline
☐ E   trimethoprim

2   On discharge Mrs M has some questions about when to take her rheumatoid arthritis medicines. Which of the following counselling points would lead to suboptimal treatment?

☐ A   Take methotrexate on the same day every week, and take folic acid the day before methotrexate.

☐ B   Take methotrexate on the same day every week, and take folic acid on the same day as methotrexate.

☐ C   Take methotrexate on the same day every week, and take folic acid the day after methotrexate.

☐ D   Take methotrexate on the same day every week, and take the folic acid two days after methotrexate.

☐ E   Take methotrexate on the same day every week, and take the folic acid on any day that is different to the methotrexate.

3   Mr B is a patient on your ward who has been admitted with hyperglycaemia. Which of his medicines is most likely to cause the fluctuation in blood glucose levels?

☐ A   aspirin
☐ B   bendroflumethiazide
☐ C   paracetamol
☐ D   ramipril
☐ E   tramadol

4   With regard to continuing professional development records, which of the following is not true?

☐ A   You can start at any point of the cycle.

☐ B   At least one third must start at reflection.

☐ C   Continuing professional development (CPD) records must be submitted online.

☐ D   The General Pharmaceutical Council (GPhC) may request to see your portfolio of evidence.

☐ E   Poor CPD records will not result in your removal from the register.

Questions 5 and 6 concern the following scenario:

Mrs D has been admitted to your gastroenterology ward with a peptic ulcer, which is currently being treated. She has a history of arthritis and myocardial infarction.

5 Which one of her regular medicines is most likely to have caused the peptic ulcer?

    ☐ A   clopidogrel 75 mg daily
    ☐ B   naproxen 250 mg twice daily
    ☐ C   propranolol 80 mg twice daily
    ☐ D   ramipril 5 mg daily
    ☐ E   simvastatin 40 mg daily

6 The medical team wants to prescribe a proton pump inhibitor alongside her regular medication. Which of the following would be most appropriate?

    ☐ A   esomeprazole
    ☐ B   lansoprazole
    ☐ C   omeprazole
    ☐ D   any of the above
    ☐ E   none of the above

7 Mrs F comes to your pharmacy asking to speak to you. She has run out of her Microgynon pill. It is Friday night and she will not be able to obtain a prescription before Monday. You decide to give her an emergency supply after interviewing her. How many tablets do you give her?

    ☐ A   3
    ☐ B   5
    ☐ C   7
    ☐ D   14
    ☐ E   21

8 Miss P comes to your pharmacy complaining of nausea. On questioning, she tells you that she is four weeks pregnant. Which of the following would be the most appropriate course of action?

    ☐ A   supply cyclizine
    ☐ B   supply *Gaviscon Advance*
    ☐ C   supply ginger tablets
    ☐ D   supply *Phenergan* (promethazine)
    ☐ E   none of the above

9   Mrs S comes into your pharmacy complaining of a sore throat, which she has had for three days. While interviewing her about her sore throat you find out that she has had some Tunes, which only gave temporary relief. She would like you to suggest an over-the-counter (OTC) remedy for her. You ask her if she is on any other medication and she tells you that she takes carbimazole 5 mg daily and propranolol 10 mg three times daily, for hyperthyroidism. Which of the following is the most appropriate advice for this patient?

☐ A   Gargle with dispersible aspirin.
☐ B   Take paracetamol.
☐ C   Take simple linctus.
☐ D   Drink plenty of water as OTC products have insufficient clinical evidence.
☐ E   Refer Mrs S to her GP.

10   Mrs C asks you which medicine would be most appropriate for treating her 5-year-old son's dry cough. What do you advise?

☐ A   codeine linctus
☐ B   dextromethorphan compound mixture
☐ C   glycerin, honey, lemon and ipecacuanha linctus
☐ D   pholcodine
☐ E   simple linctus

11   Mr Y is a night security guard and comes into your pharmacy for something to treat his hay fever. He is on no other medication and is otherwise healthy. Assuming that it is appropriate to sell him an antihistamine, which one would you not recommend?

☐ A   acrivastine
☐ B   cetirizine
☐ C   chlorphenamine
☐ D   loratadine
☐ E   none of the above

12 Mrs G is a chronic alcoholic who is being discharged from your ward. Before admission she was not taking any regular medicines. You decide to contact the discharging doctor as you have some concerns about the medicines she is being discharged on. Which drug is of most concern in alcoholic patients?

☐ A amoxicillin
☐ B cefalexin
☐ C ibuprofen
☐ D lactulose
☐ E thiamine

13 Faizah is a 10-year-old patient on your paediatric surgical ward. The surgeons wish to prescribe a postoperative anti-inflammatory for her pain. Which one of the following drugs should not be prescribed for Faizah?

☐ A aspirin
☐ B diclofenac
☐ C ibuprofen
☐ D ketorolac
☐ E none of the above should be prescribed

14 You have recently started working with another pharmacist but have some serious concerns about their behaviour and performance. You believe that patient care may be put at risk. Which of the following should you not do when initially raising your concerns?

☐ A keep a record
☐ B maintain confidentiality
☐ C report to your supervisor
☐ D report to the other pharmacist's supervisor
☐ E report to the GPhC

Questions 15 and 16 concern Mr E who has been admitted to the emergency department with suspected digoxin toxicity.

15 Which of the following is not an effect of digoxin toxicity?

☐ A confusion
☐ B hallucination
☐ C insomnia
☐ D visual disturbances
☐ E vomiting

16 You check the patient's urea and electrolytes to establish why this may be happening. Which of the following electrolyte imbalances can precipitate digoxin toxicity?

    ☐ A   hyperkalaemia
    ☐ B   hypokalaemia
    ☐ C   hypermagnesaemia
    ☐ D   hypernatraemia
    ☐ E   hyponatraemia

Questions 17 and 18 concern Mrs R, a patient with rheumatoid arthritis.

17 During your ward round Mrs R expresses concern about the side-effects of a new drug that she has been prescribed. She has recently been prescribed piroxicam. Which of the following is not a listed side-effect of this drug?

    ☐ A   diarrhoea
    ☐ B   nausea
    ☐ C   renal failure
    ☐ D   pupil dilation
    ☐ E   bleeding

18 The medical team diagnose Mrs R with mild depression as a result of her rheumatoid arthritis. The house officer asks you for some advice on what action to take. Assuming her rheumatoid arthritis is being appropriately treated, which of the following would be the best course of action?

    ☐ A   Mrs R should be offered amitriptyline
    ☐ B   Mrs R should be offered citalopram
    ☐ C   Mrs R should be offered paroxetine
    ☐ D   Mrs R should be offered cognitive behavioural therapy
    ☐ E   none of the above

19 Mrs K gives you a veterinary prescription. It is for *Otomax* (gentamicin compound) ear drops for her pet dog Parsnip, which has an ear infection. You find out that Otomax is licensed for the treatment of acute external otitis in dogs. Which of the following particulars does not legally need to be written on the prescription?

    ☐ A   qualification of the prescriber
    ☐ B   name/identification of the animal to be treated
    ☐ C   species of the animal to be treated
    ☐ D   name and address of the animal's owner
    ☐ E   statement that the drug was prescribed under the veterinary cascade

20 An inspector from the GPhC has come to inspect your pharmacy premises. He asks to see your controlled drugs registers. You have a register with the last date of entry on 26th April 2014. On which date can you dispose of the register?

    □ A   26th April 2015
    □ B   26th April 2016
    □ C   26th April 2017
    □ D   26th April 2019
    □ E   26th April 2024

21 You are accuracy checking a prescription for Mrs B. Below is a label that your dispenser has prepared.

> 28 Amiodarone 200 mg tablets
>
>
> Mrs B   1 June 2014
> **Keep out of sight and reach of children**

Which cautionary label is missing?

    □ A   Protect your skin from sunlight – even on a bright but cloudy day. Do not use sunbeds.

    □ B   This medicine may colour your urine. This is harmless.

    □ C   This medicine may make you sleepy. If this happens, do not drive or use tools or machines.

    □ D   Do not take anything containing aspirin while taking this medicine.

    □ E   Swallow this medicine whole. Do not chew or crush.

22 You are working in a hospital manufacturing unit and are having a discussion with one of the technicians about sterilisation methods. Which of the following is not classed as a method of terminal sterilisation?

   ☐ A dry heat sterilisation
   ☐ B filtration sterilisation
   ☐ C gas sterilisation
   ☐ D ionising radiation sterilisation
   ☐ E steam sterilisation

23 Continuing professional development occurs through various activities. Which of the following count towards CPD?

   ☐ A work shadowing
   ☐ B reading
   ☐ C learning by doing
   ☐ D staff training
   ☐ E all of the above

24 Mrs Y comes to your pharmacy one afternoon asking for some advice. Her 7-year-old daughter has had two small episodes of diarrhoea that morning and would like something to treat it. Her daughter is otherwise well and there are no immediate warning signs. What is the most appropriate course of action?

   ☐ A supply loperamide
   ☐ B supply *Pepto-Bismol*
   ☐ C supply oral rehydration sachets
   ☐ D advise on increased fluid intake
   ☐ E none of the above

25 Mr P comes to your pharmacy with a prescription for some temazepam tablets. You check the date on the prescription and do not dispense it as the prescription is invalid. For how long are prescriptions for temazepam valid?

   ☐ A 4 weeks
   ☐ B 8 weeks
   ☐ C 12 weeks
   ☐ D 20 weeks
   ☐ E 24 weeks

26 Mr A comes to your pharmacy with a prescription for some diazepam 5 mg tablets. You decide not to dispense the prescription as the dosing instructions are missing. Which of the following would not be acceptable on this prescription?

    ☐ A   one as directed
    ☐ B   one each night
    ☐ C   one when required
    ☐ D   once daily
    ☐ E   none of the above

27 Which schedules of controlled drugs do not allow repeats on an NHS prescription?

    ☐ A   Schedule 2 and Schedule 3
    ☐ B   Schedule 2 and Schedule 4
    ☐ C   Schedule 3 and Schedule 4
    ☐ D   Schedule 2 and Schedule 5
    ☐ E   Schedule 3 and Schedule 5

28 Mr D has been diagnosed with cellulitis and requires oral antibacterial therapy to treat it. The senior house officer asks for your advice on the ward round with regard to choice of the antibacterial. You check the patient's notes and find out that the patient has a history of anaphylaxis with penicillin. Which of the following drugs would be most suitable?

    ☐ A   cefalexin
    ☐ B   clarithromycin
    ☐ C   co-amoxiclav
    ☐ D   flucloxacillin
    ☐ E   meropenem

Questions 29–32 concern Mr H, a 51-year-old Caucasian gentleman, who has just been diagnosed with hypertension.

29 Which of the following would be the most appropriate first line treatment for Mr H's hypertension?

    ☐ A   bendroflumethiazide
    ☐ B   candesartan
    ☐ C   nifedipine
    ☐ D   ramipril
    ☐ E   verapamil

30 Mr H's GP decides he should be initiated on lisinopril 10 mg once daily. Which time of day would you advise Mr H to take his first dose of lisinopril?

    ☐ A   in the morning before breakfast
    ☐ B   in the morning with or after breakfast
    ☐ C   in the evening
    ☐ D   at night, before going to bed
    ☐ E   none of the above

31 While advising Mr H on when to take the lisinopril, he wants to know what the main side-effects of the drug are. Which of the following is a side-effect of lisinopril?

    ☐ A   hyperthyroidism
    ☐ B   persistent dry cough
    ☐ C   sleep disturbance
    ☐ D   taste disturbance
    ☐ E   micro-deposits in the eye

32 Mr H is also prescribed atorvastatin 10 mg tablets. The GP's instruction is to 'take one tablet once a day'. Mr H asks you when he should take the tablet, what do you advise?

    ☐ A   take in the morning
    ☐ B   take in the afternoon
    ☐ C   take in the evening
    ☐ D   any of the above
    ☐ E   none of the above

33 A man comes to your pharmacy complaining of diarrhoea, which started that morning. After interviewing him, you find out that he has just returned from a business trip to Laos. Which one of the following is the most appropriate course of action?

    ☐ A   supply loperamide
    ☐ B   supply *Dioralyte*
    ☐ C   supply *Pepto-Bismol*
    ☐ D   counsel on non-drug management
    ☐ E   refer to GP

34 A pharmacist's role is to enable patients and the NHS to get the most from their medicines. Which of the following is not an aspect of Medicines Optimisation?

    ☐ A   performing health checks
    ☐ B   undertaking MURs
    ☐ C   completing yellow card reports
    ☐ D   reducing polypharmacy
    ☐ E   improving inhaler technique

Questions 35 and 36 are concerning Mrs F, a patient on your general medical ward who is currently taking furosemide 40 mg o.d.

35 Mrs F is still showing signs of oedema and the medical team want to prescribe an additional diuretic. You decide to check Mrs F's urea and electrolyte results, which are as follows:

sodium 137 mmol/L (normal range, 133–145 mmol/L)
potassium 3.1 mmol/L (3.5–5.3 mmol/L)
phosphate 0.84 mmol/L (0.8–1.4 mmol/L)
urea 3.4 mmol/L (2.5–6.5 mmol/L)

Which one of the following drugs would you recommend to the doctor to add to her regimen?

    ☐ A   amiloride
    ☐ B   bendroflumethiazide
    ☐ C   bumetanide
    ☐ D   cyclopenthiazide
    ☐ E   none of the above

36 The following week Mrs F's oedema has become worse but her electrolyte levels are in range. The medical team decide to increase the furosemide dose from 40 mg once a day to 40 mg twice a day. Mrs F says that she will take her first dose in the morning as usual, but is not sure when to take the second dose. What do you advise?

    ☐ A   with her morning dose
    ☐ B   at lunchtime
    ☐ C   with her evening meal
    ☐ D   at bedtime
    ☐ E   the prescription is incorrect and needs to go back to the prescriber

37 Mr A is a patient on your ward. Recently he has developed an acute exacerbation of gout. The medical team think that it may have been precipitated by one of his medicines. Below is a list of Mr A's medication. Which one of his regular medicines do you think could have precipitated the gout?

    ☐ A   allopurinol
    ☐ B   atenolol
    ☐ C   bendroflumethiazide
    ☐ D   clopidogrel
    ☐ E   enalapril

38 With regard to controlled drug legislation, which of the following particulars does not need be recorded in the registers?

    ☐ A   drug formulation
    ☐ B   date supplied
    ☐ C   quantity supplied
    ☐ D   running balance
    ☐ E   all of the above must be recorded

39 You are a medicines information pharmacist for a hospital and have just received a query from one of the ward pharmacists. They have a patient on the ward who has brought in their own medicines from Spain. All the medicines have brand names but not the generic names. The ward pharmacist wants to know the generic names so that they can be prescribed on the drug chart. Which reference source would you initially use?

    ☐ A   *British National Formulary*
    ☐ B   *Martindale: The Complete Drug Reference*
    ☐ C   *Electronic Medicines Compendium*
    ☐ D   *British Pharmacopoeia*
    ☐ E   *European Pharmacopoeia*

40 Mr Y comes into your pharmacy with a veterinary prescription for his pet cat, Archimedes. The medicine is not licensed for use in cats and has duly been prescribed under the veterinary cascade. Which of the following particulars does not need to appear on the dispensing label?

    ☐ A   address of the prescriber
    ☐ B   name of the prescriber
    ☐ C   name/identification of the animal
    ☐ D   address of the animal's owner
    ☐ E   name of the animal's owner

41 Many drugs are stored in a refrigerator because of the increased stability this affords them. What is the recommended temperature range for such a refrigerator?

    ☐ A   0–4°C
    ☐ B   1–8°C
    ☐ C   2–8°C
    ☐ D   2–4°C
    ☐ E   2–6°C

42 You are on a post-take ward round with the medical team who are discussing Mr G, who currently takes Priadel (lithium carbonate) 400 mg daily and zopiclone 7.5mg at night when required. The medical team request lithium levels to confirm their diagnosis of suspected lithium toxicity. Which of the following is not a sign/symptom of lithium toxicity?

    ☐ A   blurred vision
    ☐ B   convulsions
    ☐ C   depression
    ☐ D   lack of coordination
    ☐ E   muscle weakness

Questions 43 and 44 regard Mr U who has recently been diagnosed with type II diabetes. He was unable to control his blood glucose levels solely with diet.

43 Mr U's GP would like to initiate an antihyperglycaemic drug. You confirm the patient's history and find out that he is taking no other medication and that he has no other illnesses. Which drug would be most appropriate for this patient?

    ☐ A   glibenclamide
    ☐ B   gliclazide
    ☐ C   insulin
    ☐ D   metformin
    ☐ E   rosiglitazone

44 During your conversation with Mr U's GP you discuss the side-effects and contraindications of each drug. Which of the following is not a side-effect of metformin?

    ☐ A   anorexia
    ☐ B   hypokalaemia
    ☐ C   low vitamin B_{12} levels
    ☐ D   metallic taste
    ☐ E   nausea

45 A local GP wants to prescribe Viagra for one of his patients who has erectile dysfunction and also diabetes. He telephones you to confirm whether he can prescribe this for his patient and you agree that he can. You remind him to add a special endorsement next to the sildenafil on the prescription, otherwise you cannot dispense it. Which endorsement do you ask him to add?

    ☐ A   Advisory Committee on Borderline Substances
    ☐ B   Brand Name
    ☐ C   British Approved Name
    ☐ D   Original Pack
    ☐ E   Selected List Scheme

46 Mrs L is taking amitriptyline for her depression. While performing an MUR you decide to discuss the side-effects of amitriptyline. Which of the following is not a side-effect of this drug?

    ☐ A   blurred vision
    ☐ B   dry mouth
    ☐ C   hypernatraemia
    ☐ D   sedation
    ☐ E   urinary retention

47 You are dispensing morphine for Mr Z's chronic pain and decide to offer him some counselling about side-effects. Which of the following is not a side-effect of morphine?

    ☐ A   constipation
    ☐ B   hypothyroidism
    ☐ C   nausea
    ☐ D   respiratory depression
    ☐ E   sedation

48 A senior house officer wishes to prescribe atenolol for one of your patients. You tell the doctor that the patient is diabetic and atenolol should be used with caution in this group of patients. What is the reason for this?

☐ **A** may affect the patient's renal function
☐ **B** may mask the symptoms of hypoglycaemia
☐ **C** may affect the patient's hepatic function
☐ **D** may elevate the patient's blood glucose levels
☐ **E** may cause bronchospasm

49 You are attending a ward round and notice that propranolol is prescribed for one of your asthma patients. You contact the prescriber and advise her to change the drug to another antihypertensive as propranolol is contraindicated in asthmatics. Which of the following is the correct explanation for the contraindication?

☐ **A** propranolol may cause bronchospasm
☐ **B** propranolol may cause bronchodilation
☐ **C** antiasthma drugs cause hypertension
☐ **D** propranolol interacts with all antiasthma drugs
☐ **E** none of the above

50 Mr T comes to see you at your anticoagulant clinic. You check the patient's INR and discover that it is higher than it should be. You read the patient's recent notes and find out that it is caused by a drug that has been recently started. Which of the following drugs could cause an increase in the patient's INR?

☐ **A** amiodarone
☐ **B** carbamazepine
☐ **C** phenobarbital
☐ **D** rifampicin
☐ **E** St John's wort

51 A customer comes to your pharmacy wanting to buy St John's wort. You ask her if she is on any other medication and she tells you that she is also taking digoxin. You decide not to sell her the tablets as the two drugs interact. What is the mechanism of the interaction?

☐ **A** digoxin increases plasma levels of St John's wort
☐ **B** St John's wort causes bradycardia
☐ **C** St John's wort decreases plasma levels of digoxin
☐ **D** digoxin inhibits the metabolism of St John's wort
☐ **E** St John's wort inhibits the metabolism of digoxin

52 Miss Wood brings in a prescription for the following:

Dianette 1 daily
Sig 2 OP

How many charges will you take from this patient?

☐ **A**   none
☐ **B**   one
☐ **C**   two
☐ **D**   three
☐ **E**   four

53 Mr L comes to your pharmacy complaining of a cold sore. After questioning him, you decide to sell him some *Zovirax* (aciclovir) topical cream. How often should he apply the cream?

☐ **A**   once a day
☐ **B**   twice a day
☐ **C**   three times a day
☐ **D**   four times a day
☐ **E**   five times a day

MULTIPLE COMPLETION QUESTIONS

Amar Iqbal

> Each of the questions or incomplete statements in this section is followed by three responses. For each question, ONE or MORE of the responses is/are correct. Decide which of the responses is/are correct, then choose:
>
> A   if 1, 2 and 3 are correct
> B   if 1 and 2 only are correct
> C   if 2 and 3 only are correct
> D   if 1 only is correct
> E   if 3 only is correct

Summary				
A	B	C	D	E
1, 2, 3	1, 2 only	2, 3 only	1 only	3 only

Questions 1–4 concern Child F, a 6-year-old girl, who presents to hospital with signs of acute severe asthma.

1   Which of the following drug(s) will be required in the ambulance or emergency area prior to admission to a hospital ward?

☐ 1   adrenaline
☐ 2   short-acting beta agonist
☐ 3   oxygen

2   You are reviewing arterial blood gas results for Child F who is now being treated for acute severe asthma. Some of the results are as follows:

sodium   140 mmol/L
potassium   3.0 mmol/L
oxygen saturation   92%

Which drug(s) is/are most likely to have contributed to the above result(s)?

☐ 1   aminophylline
☐ 2   prednisolone
☐ 3   salbutamol

3   Upon speaking to Child F's mum you find out that she normally has great difficulty using the salbutamol inhaler. You provide counselling on correct inhaler technique. On follow-up the next day, you note that the child is still having difficulty with her salbutamol inhaler. Which of the following options is/are most suitable in this case?

  □ 1   Prescribe salbutamol syrup in place of the salbutamol inhaler.
  □ 2   Ask the doctor to counsel Child F on correct inhaler technique.
  □ 3   Provide an appropriate spacer device for use with the inhaler.

4   Child F's mum would like you to counsel her on the potential side-effects of salbutamol inhaler. Which of the listed side-effects is/are a consequence of salbutamol use?

  □ 1   behavioural disturbances
  □ 2   headaches
  □ 3   fine tremors

Questions 5–7 concern controlled drugs (CDs) legislation, and the supply and record requirements for such drugs.

5   With respect to legal requirements for CDs, which of the following rows is/are correct?

	Schedule 1	Schedule 2	Schedule 3	Schedule 4	Schedule 5
1 Handwriting	Y	Y	N	N	N
2 Safe custody	Y	Y	Y	N	N
3 CD register entry required	Y	Y	N	N	N

6   Which of the following is/are true with respect to FP10 prescriptions for schedule 2 CDs?

  □ 1   The prescription for the CD should be written or typed in indelible ink.
  □ 2   The dose of the prescribed CD must be specified on the prescription.
  □ 3   The prescription for the CD is valid for 30 days from the date shown.

7 Which of the following need to be legally specified on a community pharmacy requisition for a schedule 2 controlled drug?

☐ 1 date that the requisition has been written
☐ 2 name and address of the person requisitioning the drug
☐ 3 name, strength and form of the requisitioned drug

Questions 8–11 concern over-the-counter supplies of medication to various customers who present to your chemist during a busy week.

8 Mrs CM takes *Buscopan* (hyoscine butylbromide) tablets for occasional abdominal cramps that she suffers from. What are the side-effects she is most likely to encounter with these tablets?

☐ 1 blurred vision
☐ 2 constipation
☐ 3 dry mouth

9 Mr JW regularly purchases cimetidine tablets for heartburn. He recently left hospital on some new tablets and he is unsure whether he can take cimetidine with them. Which of Mr JW's medication(s) may interact with cimetidine?

☐ 1 aspirin
☐ 2 clopidogrel
☐ 3 digoxin

10 You receive several requests for the sale of ibuprofen during the week. To which of the following patient(s) would you not sell ibuprofen over-the-counter?

☐ 1 Mr KP who regularly uses beclometasone inhaler for his asthma.
☐ 2 Mr ST who takes methotrexate for his rheumatoid arthritis.
☐ 3 Ms JN who takes lithium for her bipolar disorder.

11 Which of the following formulation(s) is/are classed as 'GSL' medicines?

☐ 1 *Acriflex* cream
☐ 2 *Cetavlex* cream
☐ 3 *Slow Sodium* tablets

Questions 12–15 concern the principles of good dispensing practice in relation to community pharmacy.

12 You receive an FP10 prescription for Mr KS who is 53 years of age. Before you can legally dispense the prescription, which of the following requirements must be fulfilled?

☐ **1** The prescription must state the name, form, and strength where appropriate of the prescribed drug.

☐ **2** The prescription must state the quantity of drug to supply or the number of days' treatment

☐ **3** The prescription must specify the age and/or date of birth of the patient.

13 The labelling machine has broken down and the technician has to handwrite a label for an item he has just dispensed, as shown below. In terms of legality, what is missing from the label?

☐ **1** address of the patient
☐ **2** cautionary and warning labels
☐ **3** 'keep out of reach of children'

56 Nicorandil tablets 20 mg		
Take ONE tablet twice daily as directed		
Mr A Dhillon 12/02/15		
Another Chemist, 7 High Street, Anytown	D	C

14 Mrs MG has brought into your chemist a carrier bag full of medication belonging to her mum who has recently passed away. The medicines are unopened and are all within their expiry date. According to the code of standards, returned medicines should:

☐ **1** be returned to stock and re-dispensed if they are in good condition
☐ **2** be recorded somewhere other than the POM register
☐ **3** not be stored in a part of the pharmacy to which the public has access.

15 While working as a locum community pharmacist you realise that you have dispensed hydralazine instead of hydroxyzine for a patient who had come to the pharmacy half an hour ago. You try to find out the patient's telephone number but you are told by directory enquiries that the number is ex-directory. You then call the operator on 100 to connect you. Which of the following is/are criteria for connection?

☐ **1** You must be calling from a community pharmacy.
☐ **2** You must explain the reason for emergency connection.
☐ **3** You must provide your name and GPhC registration number.

Questions 16–19 concern the rules governing emergency supplies of medication.

16 Which of the following healthcare professional(s) is/are allowed to request an emergency supply of a 'POM' from your chemist?

☐ **1** community practitioner nurse
☐ **2** community dentist
☐ **3** general practitioner

17 Miss LS, a regular customer in your pharmacy for the past two years comes to you on a Friday night asking for an emergency supply of the oral contraceptive pill, *Microgynon*, as she has run out. An emergency supply can be made provided:

☐ **1** you have personally interviewed her
☐ **2** she has been on *Microgynon* in the last 6 months
☐ **3** she is able to furnish a prescription within 72 hours.

18 Mr GR is flying out on holiday and presents to your pharmacy within the local airport on a Monday morning. He requests an emergency supply of atenolol 50 mg tablets as he has just checked his backpack and realised he has inadvertently left his own supply at home. He has a copy of his repeat prescription slip with him, which confirms he is on the medication. Which of the following is/are valid reasons for you to provide a supply of this drug?

☐ 1 There is an immediate need for Mr GR to have the medication.
☐ 2 On balance of risk/benefit you feel it is appropriate to ethically supply the drug.
☐ 3 The GPhC standards of conduct and ethics specify that you are responsible for your actions and omissions.

19 You are labelling an emergency supply of nifedipine 5 mg capsules made at the request of a patient. Which of the following must be legally displayed on the label?

☐ 1 the patient's name and address
☐ 2 the words 'keep out of the reach of children'
☐ 3 the words 'emergency supply'

Questions 20–23 concern the side-effect profile of commonly used prescription medication.

20 While handing out a prescription in your pharmacy for beclometasone 100 mcg inhaler (at a dose of 2 puffs b.d.) you counsel the patient on the inhaler. Which of the following is suitable advice to give?

☐ 1 Do not stop taking unless advised by your doctor.
☐ 2 Carry your steroid card with you at all times.
☐ 3 Rinse your mouth well after using this product.

21 A patient on your ward is prescribed amlodipine 10 mg tablets. Which of the following are known side-effects of this product that the patient must be made aware of?

☐ 1 flushing
☐ 2 oedema
☐ 3 myalgia

22 One of your regular customers comes to your pharmacy and requests *Piriton* (chlorphenamine) syrup for his hayfever symptoms. He asks you to explain the possible side-effects of the medication that he should be aware of. Which of the following should you tell him about?

☐ 1   drowsiness
☐ 2   dry mouth
☐ 3   taste disturbances

23 A patient who has been prescribed some metronidazole by his dentist presents to your pharmacy for you to fulfil the prescription. You advise him of an adverse drug reaction that can be caused by:

☐ 1   concomitantly taking his regular medicine, which contains 20% ethanol as an excipient
☐ 2   gargling and/or rinsing his mouth with an alcohol containing mouthwash in the morning
☐ 3   concomitantly smoking throughout the day while on the metronidazole.

Questions 24 and 25 concern the reporting of adverse reactions.

24 For which of the following is it necessary to report adverse reactions?

☐ 1   a known reaction to any medication that results in hospitalisation
☐ 2   a reaction to any medication in children
☐ 3   a reaction to a medical device

25 Mrs TH, a regular patient of yours, has just been started on *Dianette* (co-cyprindiol) for acne. When you look the drug up in the *British National Formulary*, you notice that it has a symbol next to it. What does this symbol denote?

☐ 1   All adverse drug reactions to this drug must be reported.
☐ 2   The drug is relatively new to the market and is intensively monitored.
☐ 3   The yellow card system must be utilised for this drug.

26 Which of the following is true with regard to codeine phosphate 25 mg/5mL oral solution?

☐ 1   It is not licensed in children less than 12 years of age.
☐ 2   It is cautioned in those with respiratory problems.
☐ 3   It is an opioid analgesic that can cause constipation.

27 Which of the following drug(s) for the given indication may be supplied as an emergency supply at the request of a patient?

☐ 1   morphine sulfate 10 mg/5 mL oral solution for breakthrough pain
☐ 2   naproxen 250 mg e/c tablets for inflammatory arthritic pain
☐ 3   phenobarbital 30 mg tablets for the treatment of epilepsy

28 You are researching as part of your continuing professional development (CPD) into drugs which can affect thyroid functionality. Which of the following drug(s) can affect thyroid function tests?

☐ 1   aminophylline
☐ 2   amiodarone
☐ 3   amitriptylline

29 Mrs JM, a 53-year-old, is due to start taking colchicine for an acute attack of gout. She is also on allopurinol (300 mg o.d.). Which of the following statements is/are true regarding use of these agents in acute gout?

☐ 1   Allopurinol can exacerbate acute attacks of gout and should be stopped in Mrs JM.
☐ 2   Once the colchicine course is complete it should not be repeated within 3 days.
☐ 3   Colchicine can cause diarrhoea, which will necessitate its discontinuation

30 You are reviewing the drug history of a patient who has presented to the gastroenterology ward with a stomach ulcer. Which of the following drug(s) is/are the most likely cause of the ulcer?

☐ 1   ketoprofen
☐ 2   prednisolone
☐ 3   ranitidine

31 Mr AH takes methotrexate for psoriasis. Which of the following drug(s) can potentially interact with his methotrexate?

☐ 1   aspirin
☐ 2   ibuprofen
☐ 3   paracetamol

32 Mrs SP has been prescribed lithium for manic depressive illness and is also on various other medications.
Which of the following drugs(s) interact(s) with her prescribed lithium?

☐ 1   carbamazepine
☐ 2   ibuprofen
☐ 3   flucloxacillin

33 In which of the following circumstances can information about a patient be disclosed without their consent?

☐ 1   to a coroner's court
☐ 2   to a parent of a teenager
☐ 3   to a patient's married partner

34 A father comes to your pharmacy to buy some hydrocortisone cream for his 14-year-old son. He has areas of patchy dry, itchy skin on the reverse of both of his hands. After interviewing the father, you decide to sell him the cream. Which of the following is/are suitable counselling points when supplying this product?

☐ 1   One fingertip unit of cream is sufficient to cover the back of both hands.
☐ 2   Do not apply the cream to areas of broken skin.
☐ 3   Do not use for longer than seven days without seeking medical advice.

35 Pharmacokinetic or pharmacodynamic drug interactions can occur when two or more drugs are given concurrently. Which of the following is/are significant drug interaction(s)?

☐ 1   cyclizine and ranitidine
☐ 2   lithium and naproxen
☐ 3   warfarin and amiodarone

36 You work in an independent pharmacy where baby milks and infant formula products are sold. Your manager asks you to promote the infant formulas as sales were low in the last month. Which of the following activities is/are prohibited at any place where infant formula is sold by retail?

☐ 1   Advertising of the baby milks and infant formula product.
☐ 2   Provision of free samples and discounting of these products.
☐ 3   Special displays designed to promote sales of these products.

37 A middle-aged man asks you for some advice. He has recently started taking some new medications for reflux and neuropathic pain. Since starting them, he has developed diarrhoea. He would like to know which of his medication(s) is/are most likely to cause this effect.

☐ 1 magnesium trisilicate mixture
☐ 2 morphine sulfate oral solution
☐ 3 tramadol capsules

38 Mr JG has been newly started on an angiotensin-converting enzyme inhibitor (ACEI). You are to counsel him on this class of drug. Which of the following is/are suitable advice to give when initiating treatment with an ACEI?

☐ 1 The ACEI is started at a low dose initially and then titrated depending on response.
☐ 2 ACEIs can occasionally cause a persistent irritating cough as a class side-effect.
☐ 3 The first dose is given in the morning due to the risk of postural hypotension.

39 You are operating a New Medicines Service (NMS) in your community pharmacy. Which of the following statements is/are applicable to this service?

☐ 1 The request for this service must come from the patient.
☐ 2 The service is only for newly started medicines initiated in hospital.
☐ 3 Either an NMS or MUR can be undertaken, and not both on a single patient.

40 Mr SM, a 53-year-old presents to hospital with increasing pain in his knee over a period of two months. A routine X-ray scan suggests an atypical femoral fracture and Mr SM is transferred to an orthopaedic ward. Which of the following long-term medicine(s) he is taking is/are most likely to have caused his admission?

☐ 1 omeprazole
☐ 2 quinine sulfate
☐ 3 ranitidine

41 Mr PT is prescribed some atropine eye drops to be used off-label in controlling one of his Parkinson's disease symptoms. You recall from your pharmacology lectures at university that atropine is an antimuscarinic agent. Which of the following symptoms may be alleviated by this drug?

☐ 1   dry mouth
☐ 2   constipation
☐ 3   hypersalivation

42 Mr IR, a regular patient of yours, presents a prescription for warfarin for the first time. When handing out the medicine, you counsel him. Which of the following counselling point(s) is/are correct with regard to warfarin?

☐ 1   Avoid sudden dietary changes as this may affect warfarin's clinical action.
☐ 2   Avoid alcohol as this can enhance the action of warfarin leading to possible bleeding.
☐ 3   Report any bruising or bleeding to a doctor as this will need further investigation.

43 One of your patients on the ward has recently developed severe hyponatraemia. You decide to rule out the possibility of a drug cause for this electrolyte disturbance. Which of the following drug(s) can cause hyponatraemia?

☐ 1   clopidogrel
☐ 2   furosemide
☐ 3   sertraline

44 A patient is admitted to the emergency department of your hospital with possible digoxin toxicity. Which of the following is/are possible signs indicative of digoxin toxicity?

☐ 1   nausea
☐ 2   vomiting
☐ 3   tachycardia

45 A doctor on your ward would like to prescribe a beta-blocker for Mr HF who has been diagnosed with heart failure. Which of the following beta-blockers is/are licensed for use in heart failure?

☐ 1   bisoprolol
☐ 2   carvidolol
☐ 3   metoprolol

46 Which of the following statements is/are true with regard to a GP writing a private prescription for 'phenoxymethylpenicillin 250 mg tablets' for one of his patients?

☐ 1 The prescription must be written on GP surgery headed paper.
☐ 2 The GP can request for a repeat by indicating this on the private prescription.
☐ 3 A POM register entry must be made by the supplying pharmacist for this prescription.

47 With regard to computer-generated prescriptions, which of the following is/are true?

☐ 1 The prescription must be word-processed in English.
☐ 2 The prescription does not legally need a word-processed date on it.
☐ 3 Any alterations must be in the doctor's handwriting and countersigned.

48 You are presented with a prescription for 'morphine sulfate 10 mg/5 mL oral solution' by Mr HF, one of your regular patients who is a pensioner. Which of the following is/are legal requirements for the prescription?

☐ 1 age of the patient
☐ 2 quantity in words and figures
☐ 3 strength and form of the drug

49 Miss RP comes to your pharmacy asking for the 'morning after pill'. She is 17 years of age and had missed her regular oral contraceptive pill. After interviewing her you decide not to sell the product to her. From the list of the answers given by Miss RP upon interview, choose the reason(s) that directed you to this course of action.

☐ 1 She had unprotected intercourse more than 72 hours ago.
☐ 2 She has used the 'morning after pill' once before and has not had a period yet.
☐ 3 She is currently taking co-codamol 30/500 mg tablets for headaches.

50 Which of the following is/are contraindicated in patients with asthma?

☐ 1 atenolol
☐ 2 ibuprofen
☐ 3 perindopril

CLASSIFICATION QUESTIONS

Oksana Pyzik

> In this section, for each numbered question, select the one lettered option that most closely corresponds to the answer. Within each group of questions each lettered option may be used once, more than once, or not at all.

Vitamins are used for the prevention and treatment of specific deficiency states. Questions 1–5 concern the following vitamins:

- A   vitamin A
- B   vitamin C
- C   vitamin D
- D   vitamin E
- E   vitamin K

Which of these vitamins:

1   can cause xerophthalmia in deficiency states?
2   is necessary for the production of blood clotting factors?
3   is water soluble?
4   can be used for the treatment of rickets?
5   in high doses, is contraindicated in pregnancy?

Minerals are used for the prevention and treatment of certain deficiency states. Questions 6–8 concern the following minerals:

- A   calcium
- B   magnesium
- C   phosphorus
- D   iodine
- E   zinc

Which of these minerals:

6   may be deficient in severe diabetic ketoacidosis?
7   deficiency manifests as goitre?
8   is a cofactor in enzymatic reactions and is necessary for DNA and RNA synthesis?

Questions 9–12 concern the following drugs:

- A   isosorbide mononitrate
- B   ramipril
- C   timolol
- D   bisoprolol
- E   labetolol

Which of the above drugs:

9   has relative cardioselective activity?
10   may cause throbbing headache?
11   may also block alpha adrenoceptors?
12   is used topically in glaucoma?

You are the ward pharmacist at SPG Hospital NHS Trust. You are checking a patient's drug chart and need to counsel the patient on cautionary labels for the drugs they are taking.

Questions 13–17 concern the following cautionary labels:

- A   Space doses evenly throughout the day.
- B   May cause drowsiness.
- C   Do not take indigestion remedies at the same time.
- D   Swallow whole, not chewed.
- E   Protect your skin from sunlight – even on a bright but cloudy day.

Which cautionary labels apply to the following drugs:

13   *Champix* tablets
14   clarithromycin tablets
15   erythromycin coated tablets
16   metoclopramide modified-release capsules
17   doxycycline capsules

For questions 18–20, which medicine:

- A   is used for prophylaxis of venous thromboembolism post-surgery
- B   should be avoided in patients taking MAOIs
- C   is safe to use in pregnancy
- D   may increase transaminase levels
- E   is commonly associated with a sore throat

18   dabigatran etexilate

19 pseudoephedrine
20 amiodarone hydrochloride

Questions 21–24 concern the following cautionary labels:

A Do not take indigestion remedies or medicines containing iron or zinc at the same time.
B Take an hour before food or on an empty stomach.
C Avoid exposure of skin to direct sunlight.
D Do not take milk, indigestion remedies, or medicines containing iron or zinc at the same time as this medication.
E Take with or after food.

All antibiotics have the extra precautionary label 'Complete the course'.

Which additional cautionary labels from the list are required for the following antibiotics?

21 penicillin V (phenoxymethylpenicillin)
22 ciprofloxacin
23 minocycline
24 flucloxacillin

Questions 25–28 concern the following possible side-effects:

A may cause hyperphosphataemia
B may cause hyperkalaemia
C may cause hypokalaemia
D may cause hypermagnesaemia
E may cause hypophosphataemia

Match the possible side-effects caused by the drugs below:

25 furosemide
26 bendroflumethiazide
27 lisinopril
28 amiloride

Questions 29–32 concern the following drugs:

A lithium
B haloperidol
C bupropion
D gabapentin
E carbamazepine

From the list, choose which drug:

29 may cause tardive dyskinesia?
30 may exacerbate a pre-existing seizure disorder?
31 is used as prophylaxis and treatment of mania?
32 may cause gingival hyperplasia?

33 Which of the following electrolyte imbalances predisposes to lithium toxicity?

    A hypernatraemia
    B hyponatraemia
    C hyperkalaemia
    D hypokalaemia
    E hypermagnesaemia

Questions 34–36 concern the following drugs:

    A aspirin
    B codeine
    C paracetamol
    D diphenhydramine
    E mefenamic acid

Which of the above drugs:

34 is associated with drowsiness?
35 is associated with Reye's syndrome in children?
36 is used to treat the symptoms of menorrhagia

Questions 37–39 concern the following drugs:

    A tetracycline
    B clindamycin
    C amiodarone
    D beclometasone
    E fluconazole

Which of the above drugs:

37 should be stopped immediately if diarrhoea occurs?
38 may develop hyperthyroidism or hypothyroidism?
39 may develop pulmonary fibrosis?

Questions 40–41 concern the following drugs:

A metronidazole
B penicillin
C ofloxacin
D clofazimine
E erythromycin

Which of the above drugs:

40 is used to treat *Clostridium difficile* infection?
41 treats anaerobic infections?

Questions 42–45 concern the following drugs:

A amiodarone
B metronidazole
C ciprofloxacin
D flucloxacillin
E minocycline

Which of the above drugs:

42 may cause phototoxic reactions?
43 should be avoided in epileptics?
44 may be used to treat acne?
45 should not be given to a patient with a history of penicillin allergy?

Questions 46–49 concern the following cold and flu remedies:

A guaifenesin
B honey and lemon
C eucalyptus
D pholcodine
E pseudoephedrine

Which of the above remedies:

46 acts as an antitussive?
47 acts as a demulcent?
48 acts as an expectorant?
49 has legal restrictions on quantity sold?

Questions 50–53 concern the following drugs:

    A   co-danthramer
    B   liquid paraffin
    C   cetylpyridinium chloride
    D   ranitidine bismuth citrate
    E   lactulose

Which of the above drugs:

50 may cause lipoid pneumonia?
51 may colour the urine red?
52 may cause brown stains on teeth?
53 can be used to treat hepatic encephalopathy?

Questions 54–55 concern the following drugs:

    A   buprenorphine
    B   phenobarbital
    C   morphine sulfate
    D   oxybutynin
    E   fentanyl

Which of the above drugs:

54 is exempt from controlled drug prescription requirements?
55 is exempt from safe-custody requirement?

56 Which of the following drugs must have a record kept in a controlled drugs register:

    A   temazepam
    B   tramadol
    C   diazepam
    D   diamorphine
    E   indometacin

Questions 57–58 concern the following drugs:

    A   terbinafine
    B   finasteride
    C   spirinolactone
    D   fluphenazine
    E   fexofenadine

Which of the above drugs:

57 is used to treat male pattern baldness?
58 is a type II alpha reductase inhibitor?

Questions 59–61 concern the following drugs:

    A   miconazole
    B   beclometasone
    C   piroxicam
    D   paracetamol
    E   dexamethasone

Which of the above drugs:

59 increases vulnerability to infection?
60 may cause thrush?
61 may be used to treat athlete's foot?

Questions 62–65 concern the following types of insulin:

    A   rapid-acting insulin
    B   long-acting insulin
    C   short-acting insulin
    D   medium- and long-acting insulin
    E   analogue mixture

Identify the type of insulin of each of the following:

62 insulin lispro
63 insulin aspart
64 insulin glargine
65 insulin detemir

STATEMENT QUESTIONS

Alistair Murray

> The questions in this section consist of a statement in the top row followed by a second statement beneath.
>
> You need to:
>
> decide whether the *first statement* is true or false
>
> decide whether the *second statement* is true or false
>
> Then choose:
>
> A if both statements are true and the second statement is *a correct explanation* of the first statement
> B if both statements are true but the second statement is *not a correct explanation* of the first statement
> C if the first statement is true but the second statement is false
> D if the first statement is false but the second statement is true
> E if both statements are false

1 **First statement**

Propranolol may cause vivid dreams

Second statement

Propranolol crosses the blood-brain barrier

2 **First statement**

Methotrexate interacts with non-steroidal anti-inflammatory drugs

Second statement

Piroxicam is a non-steroidal anti-inflammatory drug

3 **First statement**

Gliclazide is used as a first-line therapy in obese patients with type II diabetes

Second statement

Anorexia is a side-effect of gliclazide

4 **First statement**

Microgynon is an example of a combined oral contraceptive pill

Second statement

Combined oral contraceptive pills contain both oestrogen and testosterone

5 **First statement**

Patients taking fluoxetine should have their sodium levels checked

Second statement

Antidepressants may cause hyponatraemia

6 **First statement**

Aspirin may cause a peptic ulcer

Second statement

Aspirin inhibits bradykinin degradation

7 **First statement**

Patients taking atorvastatin should have their renal function checked regularly

Second statement

Statins may cause renal failure

8 **First statement**

Patients taking isoniazid for the treatment of tuberculosis may be prescribed pyridoxine concurrently

Second statement

Isoniazid may cause peripheral neuropathy

9 **First statement**

Gentamicin is given as a parenteral therapy for systemic infections

Second statement

Aminoglycosides are not usually absorbed from the gut

10 **First statement**

Gentamicin intravenous infusion can be prepared for intermittent infusion using glucose 5% infusion

Second statement

Choosing an incorrect intravenous additive could result in physical or chemical incompatibilities of the resulting product

11 **First statement**

Theophylline is a drug with a narrow therapeutic index

Second statement

In high doses, theophylline causes tachycardia

12 **First statement**

Patients with liver failure should be on a lower dose of propranolol

Second statement

Propranolol is a high-extraction-ratio drug

13 **First statement**

Furosemide can precipitate gout

Second statement

Loop diuretics may cause hypouricaemia

14 **First statement**

Patients at risk of osteoporosis should maintain an adequate intake of calcium and vitamin D

Second statement

Women taking long-tem oral corticosteroids are at an increased risk of osteoporosis

15 **First statement**

There is a drug interaction between warfarin and naproxen

Second statement

Naproxen can increase the anticoagulant effect of coumarins

16 **First statement**

Amiodarone is a potassium-sparing diuretic

Second statement

Amiodarone may cause phototoxicity

17 **First statement**

Phenytoin is used for the management of epilepsy

Second statement

Phenytoin can be used for tonic-clonic seizures

18 **First statement**

Many drugs may cause constipation

Second statement

Tramadol is a drug that may cause constipation

19 **First statement**

A patient with a fever may also have a raised level of C-reactive protein

Second statement

C-reactive protein is an inflammatory marker

20 **First statement**

Patients who require rapid digitalisation with digoxin need to be given a loading dose

Second statement

Digoxin has a very long half-life

21 **First statement**

Amiloride may induce hyperkalaemia

Second statement

Amiloride is a potassium-sparing diuretic

22 **First statement**

Patients using steroid inhalers should be counselled to rinse their mouth well after use

Second statement

The use of steroid inhalers may cause gingivitis

23 **First statement**

A patient receiving a prescription for warfarin 1 mg tablets and warfarin 3 mg tablets on the same FP10 form would have to pay one NHS prescription charge

Second statement

Different strengths of the same formulation prescribed on the same form attract only one charge

24 **First statement**

Amitriptyline can be used to treat neuropathic pain

Second statement

Amitriptyline may cause drowsiness

25 **First statement**

Bananas are a good source of potassium

Second statement

Hyperkalaemia predisposes to digoxin toxicity

26 **First statement**

Lithium interacts with paracetamol

Second statement

Paracetamol reduces the excretion of lithium

27 **First statement**

Flucloxacillin interacts with the combined oral contraceptive pill

Second statement

Flucloxacillin suppresses the gut flora

28 **First statement**

Audit is a part of clinical governance

Second statement

An audit should always lead to changes in practice

29 **First statement**

It is not possible to provide emergency hormonal contraception to a 14-year-old girl with a parent or guardian giving consent

Second statement

Levonelle One Step can only be sold to women over 16 years of age

30 **First statement**

Nicotine replacement products should only be recommended to patients who have chronic obstructive pulmonary disease (COPD) if their doctor is informed about it

Second statement

Smoking tobacco does not cause COPD but can make it worse

31 **First statement**

The GPhC can inspect a pharmacy to check that conversations cannot be heard outside of a consultation room in a pharmacy

Second statement

Premises should protect the privacy, dignity and confidentiality of patients and the public who receive pharmacy services

32 **First statement**

All pharmacy-only (P) medicines must be sold by a pharmacist registered in the UK

Second statement

Only general sales list (GSL) medicines can be sold by counter assistants or pharmacy technicians

The following questions (33–36) concern Miss L, a patient who regularly uses the pharmacy where you are working today. She has lost her prescribed medicines. It is a Saturday afternoon and her GP surgery is closed. She would like an emergency supply of her usual medications. There is not a locally-commissioned service for emergency supplies. She is also interested in the pharmacy's Stop Smoking Service. She has no other medical conditions and no family history of disease. On checking the PMR you find that she normally receives the following items:

126 × *Logynon* tablets
2 × salbutamol 100 mcg inhaler for mild asthma

33 **First statement**

It is acceptable to supply some *Logynon* tablets as an emergency supply

Second statement

An emergency supply of a prescription-only medicine can only be provided if the patient regularly uses the pharmacy where they request the supply

34 **First statement**

You should refuse to supply the *Logynon* tablets on clinical grounds

Second statement

Smoking tobacco while using a combined oral contraceptive increases the risk of arterial disease

35 **First statement**

Stopping smoking may help Miss L's asthma symptoms

Second statement

Salbutamol relaxes smooth muscle in the airways by acting on beta$_2$ adrenoceptors to relieve asthma symptoms

36 **First statement**

You should provide only three *Logynon* tablets since Miss L should be able to see her GP on Monday in order to obtain a prescription for further supply

Second statement

An emergency supply should only ever be for the exact number of days until a prescriber can issue another prescription

The following questions (37–40) concern Mr W, a 56-year-old man who lives locally and uses the pharmacy where you are working as a locum pharmacist.

Mr W has come into the pharmacy to complain that there has been an error with his prescription that he collected two days ago. He was prescribed lansoprazole 30 mg capsules and he received lansoprazole 15 mg capsules, labelled as lansoprazole 30 mg capsules. He has taken the 15 mg capsules for the past two days. He is upset about the error but does not feel unwell. Mr W would also like to buy some painkillers for a headache.

37 **First statement**

You should apologise that an error has been made

Second statement

You should find out who the responsible pharmacist was on the day that the error occurred

38 **First statement**

It is good practice to retain the incorrect medicines in the pharmacy

Second statement

Having as many details as possible about the error can help the team to understand why it happened so as to avoid it happening again

39 **First statement**

You should tell Mr W to urgently see his GP to discuss the matter

Second statement

He is likely to be experiencing life-threatening symptoms as a result of the under-dosing due to the error

40 **First statement**

Ibuprofen can be used for the treatment of a mild-to-moderate headache

Second statement

Paracetamol may be a more appropriate choice because of Mr W's medical history

The following questions (41–44) concern Mr T, a 68-year-old man, who presents an NHS prescription from a local dentist for *Augmentin* 625 mg tablets ×21 with the directions 'one tablet three times daily'. It was prescribed on the same day as he presents in the pharmacy.

41 **First statement**

You inform Mr T that it is not possible to dispense this item for him

Second statement

Dentists have to prescribe medicines generically on NHS prescriptions

42 **First statement**

You should ask Mr T if he has any drug allergies

Second statement

Arrange for an alternative medication if Mr T says he has a penicillin allergy

43 **First statement**

If Mr T returns with a prescription for co-amoxiclav 250/125 mg tablets he should pay two NHS prescription charges

Second statement

There is a prescription charge for each ingredient in compound preparations such as co-amoxiclav

44 **First statement**

You should counsel Mr T about the signs and symptoms of cholestatic jaundice

Second statement

Men over 65 are more prone to developing cholestatic jaundice due to treatment with co-amoxiclav

45 **First statement**

Pharmacists should keep at least 12 CPD entries per year (one per month) to meet the GPhC's standards

Second statement

Pharmacists should record how their CPD has contributed to the quality or development of their practice

46 **First statement**

Pregnant women should, where possible, avoid travel to areas with a high risk of malaria transmission

Second statement

Antimalarials are dangerous to the health of all pregnant women

47 **First statement**

Long-term oxygen therapy is used to treat patients with COPD who have a P_aO_2 <7.3 kPa when breathing air

Second statement

Short-burst oxygen therapy can be prescribed for patients who have breathlessness associated with COPD

48 **First statement**

Lyclear Creme Rinse is only prescribed for the treatment of scabies, not head lice

Second statement

Shampoos such as *Lyclear Creme Rinse* are not considered to be an effective treatment against head lice

49 **First statement**

Serious adverse drug reactions in children should be reported to the MHRA via the yellow card scheme

Second statement

The action and pharmacokinetics of drugs in children are the same as in adults

50 **First statement**

An adverse reaction to *Tegaderm* hydrocolloid dressings should be reported using the yellow card scheme

Second statement

Adverse reactions to medical devices, as well as medicines, should be reported to the MHRA

Calculation questions

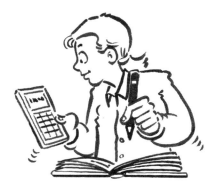

SIMPLE COMPLETION QUESTIONS

Amar Iqbal, Alistair Murray and Ryan Hamilton

> Each of the questions or statements in this section is followed by five suggested answers. Select the best answer in each situation.

1   A patient in theatre is suffering from malignant hyperthermia following anaesthesia. The anaesthetist wishes to prescribe dantrolene sodium by rapid intravenous injection. The patient weighs 70 kg. What is the collective maximum dose this patient can have?

    ☐ A   70 mg
    ☐ B   140 mg
    ☐ C   280 mg
    ☐ D   360 mg
    ☐ E   700 mg

2   A GP wants to prescribe *Gynest* cream for one of her patients. How many milligrams of estriol are there in one tube of this cream?

    ☐ A   1 mg
    ☐ B   8 mg
    ☐ C   10 mg
    ☐ D   80 mg
    ☐ E   100 mg

3   You receive a prescription for a reducing dose of prednisolone in Child H who has brittle asthma. The dose is to be reduced until Child H is back on his normal alternating daily dose. The prescribing doctor has written: '30 mg o.d. for 5 days, then 20 mg o.d. for 3 days, then 10 mg o.d. for 3 days, then 5 mg alternate days'. The prescription asks for a 28-day supply.
How many 5-mg tablets should you supply?

  ☐ A   48
  ☐ B   49
  ☐ C   52
  ☐ D   56
  ☐ E   57

4   The half-life of a new drug compound is said to be approximately 4 hours. It takes 19.6 hours to reach steady state. Approximately how many half-lives does it take the new drug compound to reach steady state?

  ☐ A   1
  ☐ B   2
  ☐ C   3
  ☐ D   4
  ☐ E   5

5   Baby K who weighs 0.84 kg requires some total parenteral nutrition (TPN). His total daily fluid intake is 100 mL/kg/day and is to consist solely of his TPN bag. The neonatal sister asks for you to check her calculated rate for the TPN that she is to set up via an infusion pump. Which of the following is the correct rate assuming you have a 250 mL stock bag of TPN available?

  ☐ A   0.84 mL/hour
  ☐ B   1.75 mL/hour
  ☐ C   3.5 mL/hour
  ☐ D   4.2 mL/hour
  ☐ E   10.4 mL/hour

6   You are asked for instructions on how to dilute solution A (1 in 100) in order to produce a 1 in 1000 solution. Which of the following is the correct dilution?

    □ A   1 part of solution A added to 9 parts diluent
    □ B   1 part of solution A added to 10 parts diluent
    □ C   1 part of solution A added to 11 parts diluent
    □ D   1 part of solution A added to 99 parts diluent
    □ E   1 part of solution A added to 100 parts diluent

7   You receive a request for omeprazole 10 mg/5mL suspension. Given that omeprazole has a molecular weight of approximately 345, how many millimoles of omeprazole are there (to one decimal place) in a 100 mL bottle of this product?

    □ A   0.06 mmol
    □ B   0.1 mmol
    □ C   0.6 mmol
    □ D   1 mmol
    □ E   6 mmol

8   Mr KF is admitted to hospital while on *Uniphyllin Continus* M/R tablets at a dose of 200 mg twice daily. Mr KF has dysphagia and so is finding it difficult to tolerate the tablets. As theophylline syrup is unlicensed and not readily available in your hospital, it is decided to switch Mr KF to aminophylline injection. What is the most suitable dose of aminophylline for Mr KF?

    □ A   80 mg
    □ B   160 mg
    □ C   240 mg
    □ D   320 mg
    □ E   400 mg

9   You are called by a neonatal nurse. She needs to make up a 500 mL bag of glucose 12% solution. She has in stock 500 mL bags of glucose 50% and glucose 10%. What approximate volume of each will she need to make up the required bag?

    □ A   315 mL of glucose 10% and 185 mL of glucose 50%
    □ B   380 mL of glucose 10% and 120 mL of glucose 50%
    □ C   440 mL of glucose 10% and 60 mL of glucose 50%
    □ D   475 mL of glucose 10% and 25 mL of glucose 50%
    □ E   490 mL of glucose 10% and 10 mL of glucose 50%

10 What is the body surface area (BSA) of Child S, a 5-year-old who weighs 18 kg and is 3 ft 8 in tall?

BSA (m^2) $= \sqrt{}$ { [height (cm) $\times$ weight (kg)] / 3600 }

    ☐ A   0.62 m^2
    ☐ B   0.65 m^2
    ☐ C   0.68 m^2
    ☐ D   0.71 m^2
    ☐ E   0.74 m^2

11 A patient is prescribed alfacalcidol at a dose of 500 nanograms three times per week. The dispensary has capsules that are half the strength of the prescribed dose. How many capsules would you supply to cover 28 days?

    ☐ A   12
    ☐ B   18
    ☐ C   24
    ☐ D   30
    ☐ E   36

12 How many *Rifater* tablets should a man weighing 70 kg be prescribed to cover the initial phase of his unsupervised treatment for tuberculosis?

    ☐ A   180
    ☐ B   240
    ☐ C   300
    ☐ D   360
    ☐ E   420

13 A child weighing 20 kg requires gentamicin 7.5 mg/kg/day. What volume of gentamicin 80 mg in 2mL should be given every 8 hours?

    ☐ A   1.25 mL
    ☐ B   2.5 mL
    ☐ C   3.75 mL
    ☐ D   7.5 mL
    ☐ E   12.5 mL

14 What weight of clobetasol propionate is present in 30 g of *Dermovate* cream?

    ☐ A   15 mg
    ☐ B   5 mg
    ☐ C   1.5 mg
    ☐ D   0.05 mg
    ☐ E   0.015 mg

15 Drug M is available as an elixir containing 150 mg/5 mL. You receive a prescription for 225 mg q.d.s. for two weeks. What is the volume that should be supplied?

    ☐ A   140 mL
    ☐ B   210 mL
    ☐ C   280 mL
    ☐ D   420 mL
    ☐ E   490 mL

16 What volume of a 20% w/v solution contains 6.6 g of ingredient?

    ☐ A   66 mL
    ☐ B   33 mL
    ☐ C   30 mL
    ☐ D   6.6 mL
    ☐ E   3.3 mL

17 Mrs D uses hypromellose 0.3% w/v eye drops to treat dry eyes. Her daily dose is one drop into both eyes five times daily. Assume that there are 15 drops/mL. How many 10 mL bottles would she be supplied with for 28 days' treatment?

    ☐ A   1.4
    ☐ B   1.87
    ☐ C   2
    ☐ D   14
    ☐ E   18.67

18 Mrs V is prescribed a course of prednisolone enteric-coated tablets with a reducing dose. Her instructions on the prescription are as follows:

> Week 1: 20 mg daily
> Week 2: 17.5 mg daily
> Week 3: 15 mg daily
> Week 4: 12.5 mg daily
> Week 5: 10 mg daily
> Week 6: 7.5 mg daily
> Weeks 7 and 8: 5 mg daily
> Weeks 9 and 10: 2.5 mg daily

How many tablets should you supply for this prescription?

- [ ] **A**   112 × 5 mg tablets and 70 × 1 mg tablets
- [ ] **B**   112 × 5 mg tablets and 28 × 2.5 mg tablets
- [ ] **C**   119 × 5 mg tablets and 88 × 1 mg tablets
- [ ] **D**   119 × 5 mg tablets and 35 × 2.5 mg tablets
- [ ] **E**   137 × 5 mg tablets

19 How much water should you use when diluting Concentrated Peppermint Water BP to produce 500 mL of Double-Strength Peppermint Water BP?

- [ ] **A**   19 mL
- [ ] **B**   25 mL
- [ ] **C**   95 mL
- [ ] **D**   250 mL
- [ ] **E**   475 mL

20 Mr F has been prescribed an oral loading dose of digoxin for rapid digitalisation. Which of the following prescriptions would give the highest appropriate dose over 24 hours to achieve this?

- [ ] **A**   10 × 250 mcg tablets
- [ ] **B**   6 × 250 mcg tablets
- [ ] **C**   10 × 125 mcg tablets
- [ ] **D**   6 × 125 mcg tablets
- [ ] **E**   20 × 62.5 mcg tablets

21 There is currently a supply problem with *Atripla* tablets and you need to continue Mr J's antiretroviral treatment with alternative products to achieve the same doses. Which of the following would be the same for 30 days' supply?

☐ A   30 × *Sustiva* 600 mg tablets and 30 × *Viread* 245 mg tablets
☐ B   30 × *Eviplera* tablets and 90 × *Sustiva* 200 mg capsules
☐ C   30 × *Truvada* tablets and 90 × *Sustiva* 200 mg capsules
☐ D   60 × *Sustiva* 200 mg capsules and 30 × *Eviplera* tablets
☐ E   30 × *Truvada* tablets and 30 × *Viread* 245 mg tablets

22 Mr E has a prescription for *Eumovate* cream from the dermatology outpatient department. The prescription indicates that Mr E will be applying the cream to the left arm for one month. Which of the following would be a suitable amount to dispense?

☐ A   60 g
☐ B   90 g
☐ C   100 g
☐ D   15 g
☐ E   200 g

Questions 23 and 24 concern the following scenario:

Mrs G comes to see you about losing weight and would like to try orlistat. During the consultation you take some weights and measurements and find that Mrs G is 4 ft 11 in tall and weighs 13 st and 1 lb.

23 What is Mrs G's body mass index (BMI) expressed as a whole number?

☐ A   19 kg/m^2
☐ B   23 kg/m^2
☐ C   37 kg/m^2
☐ D   42 kg/m^2
☐ E   56 kg/m^2

24 How much weight does Mrs G need to lose in order to reach a healthy BMI of 24 kg/m^2?

☐ A   4 st 8 lbs
☐ B   4 st 11 lbs
☐ C   5 st 1 lb
☐ D   5 st 6 lbs
☐ E   5 st 8 lbs

Question **25** concerns the following scenario:

Mr E is on your acute renal unit and the nephrology team would like to prescribe some medicines. You take a look at Mr E's admission notes and discern the following information:
Age: 60 years
Height: 1.8 m
Ideal body weight: 80 kg
Blood pressure: 150/95 mmHg
Serum potassium: 5.0 mmol/L
Serum creatinine: 200 micromol/L
Urea: 7.2 mmol/L

25 You decide to use the Cockcroft and Gault formula to calculate his renal function. What is Mr E's estimated creatinine clearance rate?

  □ **A**   30.7 mL/minute
  □ **B**   32.0 mL/minute
  □ **C**   39.4 mL/minute
  □ **D**   40.0 mL/minute
  □ **E**   41.7 mL/minute

Questions 26 and 27 concern the following scenario:

Mr V is due to commence a course of chemotherapy and the consultants would like to dose him by body surface area (BSA).

Mosteller formula for BSA

$$\text{BSA (m}^2) = ([\text{height (cm)} \times \text{weight (kg)}] / 3600)^{0.5}$$

26 You look at Mr V's notes and find that he is 1.8 m tall and weighs 80 kg. What is his body surface area?

  □ **A**   0.02 m^2
  □ **B**   2 m^2
  □ **C**   4 m^2
  □ **D**   8 m^2
  □ **E**   20 m^2

27 The consultant decides to initiate busulfan at a dose of 1.8 mg/m². What should the dose be?

  □ A 0.04 mg
  □ B 3.6 mg
  □ C 7.2 mg
  □ D 14.4 mg
  □ E 360 mg

Questions 28–30 concern the following scenario:

You are visiting a nursing home to undertake medicines reviews for the patients when you are approached by one of the medics. His patient Mrs R is currently taking *Zomorph* capsules 60 mg twice daily. However, she is starting to experience regular breakthrough pain and rescue doses of *Oramorph* at one-tenth of her total daily *Zomorph* dose are not controlling the pain sufficiently.

28 You mutually agree to increase the rescue dose of *Oramorph* to one-sixth of her total daily *Zomorph* dose. What would the dose be?

  □ A 2 mg
  □ B 4 mg
  □ C 5 mg
  □ D 10 mg
  □ E 20 mg

29 When prescribing liquids it is necessary to state the number of millilitres to give. How many millilitres of *Oramorph* would be appropriate for Mrs R to receive for each rescue dose?

  □ A 1 mL
  □ B 2.5 mL
  □ C 10 mL
  □ D 20 mL
  □ E 25 mL

30 You return to the nursing home the following week and the medical team wish to transfer Mrs R on to fentanyl patches. When you review her notes you see she is now receiving *Zomorph* 70 mg twice daily and receives one or two rescue doses of *Oramorph* at one-seventh of the daily dose each day. Which fentanyl patch would be the most appropriate to prescribe for Mrs R?

    ☐ A   fentanyl 12 mcg/hour patch
    ☐ B   fentanyl 25 mcg/hour patch
    ☐ C   fentanyl 50 mcg/hour patch
    ☐ D   fentanyl 75 mcg/hour patch
    ☐ E   fentanyl 100 mcg/hour patch

Question 31 concerns the following scenario:

Mr Q has been admitted to your ward and has had a nasogastric tube fitted. Upon taking his medication history you note he was taking phenytoin capsules 100 mg twice daily to control his epilepsy. The medical team have prescribed phenytoin liquid, which you know is not bioequivalent.

31 You find that 100 mg of phenytoin sodium is equivalent to 90 mg of the phenytoin base. How many mL of phenytoin suspension should Mr Q receive each day?

    ☐ A   6.0 mL
    ☐ B   16.6 mL
    ☐ C   18.5 mL
    ☐ D   30.0 mL
    ☐ E   33.3 mL

Question 32 concerns the following scenario:

You are a quality control pharmacist working in the QC labs for your hospital's manufacturing unit. You are testing the concentration of drug Z in a batch of solution utilising UV-visible spectrophotometry at 270 nm. Your QC department has produced the following calibration curve for drug Z.

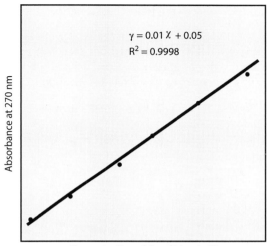

$$\gamma = 0.01\, \chi + 0.05$$
$$R^2 = 0.9998$$

Absorbance at 270 nm

Concentration of drug Z (mg/mL)

32 The UV-visible absorbance reading at 270 nm for this batch is 0.550. What is the concentration of drug Z in the solution?

☐ **A**   0.5 mg/mL
☐ **B**   5 mg/mL
☐ **C**   49.5 mg/mL
☐ **D**   50 mg/mL
☐ **E**   60 mg/mL

Question 33 concerns the following scenario:

Miss L is going travelling and her GP calls you to discuss malaria prophylaxis as she will be visiting Vietnam. Miss L will arrive in Hanoi where she will stay for a week, before heading to visit family in a rural town in South Vietnam for two weeks, then returning to the UK. You confirm that it will be unlikely for Miss L to avoid exposure to the sun so you suggest that the GP prescribes *Malarone* tablets once daily.

33 How many tablets of *Malarone* should be prescribed for Miss L?

☐ **A**   14
☐ **B**   16
☐ **C**   21
☐ **D**   23
☐ **E**   28

Questions 34 and 35 concern the following scenario:

Mr A has been admitted to your ward with a pulmonary embolism. His renal impairment prevents him from receiving enoxaparin so the medical team decides to initiate heparin, dosed by body weight. Mr A is obese so it is necessary to determine his ideal body weight (IBW).

Male IBW (kg) = 50 kg + 2.3 kg for each inch over 5 ft

34 Mr A has his height measured as 5 ft 10 in. What loading dose of heparin should he receive?

        ☐ A   1314 units
        ☐ B   3750 units
        ☐ C   5000 units
        ☐ D   5475 units
        ☐ E   10 000 units

35 It will also be necessary for Mr A to receive a continuous infusion of heparin. What dose should he receive?

        ☐ A   1314 units/hour
        ☐ B   3750 units/hour
        ☐ C   5000 units/hour
        ☐ D   5475 units/hour
        ☐ E   none of the above

Question 36 concerns the following scenario:

You are working in the microbiology lab, investigating the effectiveness of your first-line antibacterial agents against an isolated strain of *Staphylococcus aureus*. In order to report the effectiveness of these antibacterial agents you need to calculate the number of colony forming units (CFUs) per mL of the original culture. This is determined by making serial dilutions of the original culture, growing 200 microlitres of these serial dilutions on agar plates, then counting the individual CFUs. This is done in triplicate.

After incubation, you count the number of CFUs on each plate and record the following results:

Dilution factor	Colony forming units (CFUs) counted per plate		
1 in 10 000	12	10	11
1 in 1000	110	120	125
1 in 100	Confluent growth; could not count colonies		
1 in 10	Confluent growth; could not count colonies		
0 (original culture)	Confluent growth; could not count colonies		

36 What is the mean average number of CFUs (to the nearest 10) per mL in the original culture as determined by the CFU counts given above?

    ☐ A   60 000
    ☐ B   114 100
    ☐ C   114 160
    ☐ D   570 510
    ☐ E   570 830

Questions 37 and 38 concern the following scenario:

Mrs J has been prescribed intravenous vancomycin 2 g daily, in two divided doses, for the treatment of septicaemia thought to be related to her vascular catheter.

37 Assuming Mrs J is not fluid-restricted, what is the minimum volume of fluid that each dose of vancomycin should be made up to?

    ☐ A   100 mL
    ☐ B   200 mL
    ☐ C   500 mL
    ☐ D   1000 mL
    ☐ E   5000 mL

38 The nursing team plan to make up each dose of vancomycin to 200 mL. What is the maximum rate the infusion pump should be set to?

    ☐ A   0.05 mL/minute
    ☐ B   1.75 mL/minute
    ☐ C   2.00 mL/minute
    ☐ D   5.00 mL/minute
    ☐ E   20.00 mL/minute

Question 39 concerns the following scenario:

Mr B is one of your regular warfarin patients who has just attended the anticoagulation clinic. Upon inspecting his warfarin book you note he is now prescribed warfarin 3 mg and 4 mg on alternate days.

39 Assuming his next dose will be 4 mg, how many warfarin tablets do you need to supply Mr B to last him four weeks?

    ☐ **A**   100 × 1 mg tablets
    ☐ **B**   48 × 2 mg tablets
    ☐ **C**   42 × 2 mg tablets and 14 × 1 mg tablets
    ☐ **D**   28 × 3 mg tablets and 14 × 1 mg tablets
    ☐ **E**   14 × 3 mg tablets and 14 × 4 mg tablets

Questions 40 and 41 concern the following scenario:

Mrs W is 26 weeks pregnant and suffers from iron-deficiency anaemia. A trial with oral ferrous sulfate failed to produce a significant response and the medical team now want to trial Mrs W on intravenous *Venofer*.

Total iron dose (mg) = body weight (kg)

$$\times \ \{[\text{target Hb (g/dL)} - \text{actual Hb (g/dL)}] \times 2.4\} + \chi$$

where χ is the mg of iron needed to replenish iron stores.

$X = 500$ mg (or 15 mg/kg in patients weighing less than 35 kg).

40 You look in Mrs W's notes and find the following information:

Age: 32 years
Height: 5 ft 3 in
Weight before pregnancy: 58 kg
Gestation: 26 weeks
Iron: 5 micromol/L
Haemoglobin: 9.0 g/dL
Blood pressure: 130/80 mmHg

The consultant would like to aim for a haemoglobin level of 14 g/dL in Mrs W. What is the total dose of iron this patient needs?

    ☐ **A**   620 mg
    ☐ **B**   1196 mg
    ☐ **C**   3701 mg
    ☐ **D**   7460 mg
    ☐ **E**   29 696 mg

41 Each dose of *Venofer* must not exceed 200 mg and the patient should receive no more than three doses in any one week. How many doses over how many weeks should Mrs W expect to receive?

    ☐ **A**   two doses in 1 week
    ☐ **B**   three doses in 1 week
    ☐ **C**   six doses in 2 weeks
    ☐ **D**   38 doses in 13 weeks
    ☐ **E**   50 doses in 17 weeks

Questions 42 and 43 concern the following scenario:

Mr C is on your cardiology ward and requires rapid digitalisation. The medical team want to administer digoxin via the intravenous route and ask for your help in calculating the correct dose. Upon looking at his notes you retrieve the following information:
Age: 65 years
Weight: 75 kg
Height: 5 ft 5 in
Blood pressure: 150/90 mmHg
Heart rate: 123 bpm
Creatinine clearance (CrCl): 49 mL/minute

42 First you need to calculate Mr C's digoxin clearance (DigCl) rate:

DigCl (L/hour) = (0.06 × CrCl) + (0.05 × ideal body weight (kg))

Male IBW (kg) = 50 kg + 2.3 kg for each inch over 5 ft

What is Mr C's digoxin clearance rate?

    ☐ **A**   0.96 L/hour
    ☐ **B**   6.02 L/hour
    ☐ **C**   6.25 L/hour
    ☐ **D**   7.94 L/hour
    ☐ **E**   9.04 L/hour

43 Utilising Mr C's digoxin clearance rate you can estimate the dose of digoxin he will need:

$$C_{pss} = \frac{(F \times D)}{(DigCl \times t)}$$

where F is the bioavailability of the formulation, D is the dose of digoxin (mcg), t is the time interval between doses (hours), and C_{pss} is the digoxin serum level at steady state (mcg/L)

The therapeutic range of digoxin in atrial fibrillation is 1.5–2.0 mcg/L. What dose of digoxin should Mr C receive?

☐ A   50 mcg daily
☐ B   62.5 mcg daily
☐ C   125 mcg daily
☐ D   250 mcg daily
☐ E   375 mcg daily

Question 44 concerns the following scenario:

Mrs K has been admitted to your emergency department with suspected digoxin toxicity. After taking blood tests her serum digoxin level is found to be 3.0 mcg/L and the medical team want to initiate *DigiFab*. She was weighed on admission as 60 kg.

No. DigiFav vials required

$$= \frac{(patient\ weight\ (kg) \times digoxin\ level\ (micrograms/L))}{100}$$

44 How many whole vials of *DigiFab* should be used to treat Mrs K?

☐ A   1.0
☐ B   1.8
☐ C   2.0
☐ D   3.0
☐ E   3.8

Question 45 concerns the following scenario:

Ashley is a 12-year-old boy on your paediatric medical ward who has recently been receiving 10 mg methylprednisolone intravenously four times a day for severe inflammation.

45 The medical team would like to transfer Ashley on to prednisolone. What dose should initially be prescribed?

  ☐ A 1.25 mg daily
  ☐ B 10 mg daily
  ☐ C 12.5 mg daily
  ☐ D 25 mg daily
  ☐ E 50 mg daily

Question 46 concerns the following scenario:

Nashwa is a 7-year-old girl on your paediatric intensive care unit suffering from pulmonary oedema. The consultant has requested Nashwa be placed on a continuous intravenous infusion of furosemide at a dose of 0.5 mg/kg.

46 What is the minimum volume of diluent the nursing team can use when making up enough furosemide infusion to treat Nashwa for an 8-hour period?

  ☐ A 0.25 mL
  ☐ B 5.75 mL
  ☐ C 11.5 mL
  ☐ D 46 mL
  ☐ E 138 mL

Question 47 concerns the following scenario:

You are working in a hospital aseptic unit and you are asked to produce a batch of intravenous infusion bags containing 40 mmol of potassium. Atomic weight of potassium is 39.0 and chlorine is 35.5.

47 How many millilitres of concentrated potassium chloride 15% w/v need to be added to each infusion bag?

  ☐ A 0.012 mL
  ☐ B 1.15 mL
  ☐ C 10.40 mL
  ☐ D 19.87 mL
  ☐ E 29.33 mL

Question 48 concerns the following scenario:

Mr Q, who weighs 80 kg, requires an intravenous infusion of dopamine hydrochloride, which has been prescribed at a rate of 3 mcg/kg/minute. The nurses have infusion bags of 160 mg dopamine in 100 mL of glucose 5%.

48 At what rate should the infusion pump be set?

    ☐ A   0.9 mL/hour
    ☐ B   4 mL/hour
    ☐ C   6 mL/hour
    ☐ D   9 mL/hour
    ☐ E   40 mL/hour

Questions 49–52 concern the pharmaceutical compounding of non-sterile products.

49 You are asked to make a chlorhexidine solution for the disinfection of wounds and burns. What strength of chlorhexidine solution (mg/mL) do you need to prepare so that when 5 mL is diluted to 200 mL it gives a final concentration of 0.05% (w/v)?

    ☐ A   0.02 mg/mL
    ☐ B   0.2 mg/mL
    ☐ C   2 mg/mL
    ☐ D   10 mg/mL
    ☐ E   20 mg/mL

50 You have been given a prescription for 60 g of Compound Benzoic Acid Ointment BP to be applied to the affected areas twice daily. Taking into account that you will need to make a 5% excess, how much of each of the active ingredients is required to produce this ointment?

    ☐ A   3.78 g benzoic acid and 1.89 g salicylic acid
    ☐ B   3.96 g benzoic acid and 1.98 g salicylic acid
    ☐ C   37.8 g benzoic acid and 18.9 g salicylic acid
    ☐ D   39.6 g benzoic acid and 19.8 g salicylic acid
    ☐ E   60.0 g benzoic acid and 30.0 g salicylic acid

51 You have received an order for 15 g of hydrocortisone cream 2%. Your pharmacy only has the 1% and 2.5% formulations available. How much of each of these creams do you need to use in order to make the required cream?

    ☐ A   2.5 g of 1% cream and 12.5 g of 2.5% cream
    ☐ B   5 g of 1% cream and 10 g of 2.5% cream
    ☐ C   7.5 g of 1% cream and 7.5 g of 2.5% cream
    ☐ D   10 g of 1% cream and 5 g of 2.5% cream
    ☐ E   12.5 g of 1% cream and 2.5 g of 2.5% cream

52 What weight of salicylic acid powder must you add to 50 g of 2% (w/w) salicylic acid cream to produce a cream of 5% (w/w)?

    ☐ A   0.79 g
    ☐ B   1.50 g
    ☐ C   1.58 g
    ☐ D   3.00 g
    ☐ E   3.16 g

MULTIPLE COMPLETION QUESTIONS

Amar Iqbal and Alistair Murray

Each of the questions or incomplete statements in this section is followed by three responses. For each question, ONE or MORE of the responses is/are correct. Decide which of the responses is/are correct, then choose:

A   if 1, 2, and 3 are correct
B   if 1 and 2 only are correct
C   if 2 and 3 only are correct
D   if 1 only is correct
E   if 3 only is correct

Summary				
A	B	C	D	E
1, 2, 3	1, 2 only	2, 3 only	1 only	3 only

1   Which of the following contain approximately the same amount of sodium as a single 5 mL spoonful of *Gaviscon Liquid* (peppermint flavour)?

☐ 1   5 mL of *Peptac* suspension
☐ 2   5 mL of *Acidex* liquid
☐ 3   5 mL of *Gastrocote* liquid

2   Which of the following preparations at the said doses provide at least 400 units of vitamin D?

☐ 1   *Adcal-D3* caplets at a dose of 1 o.m.
☐ 2   *Calcichew-D3* caplets at a dose of 1 o.m.
☐ 3   *Natecal D3* tablets at a dose of 1 o.m.

3   Which of the following statements is/are true with regard to an intra-venous dopamine infusion that is due to be prescribed to Baby B, a preterm baby of 28 weeks' gestation who weighs 0.9 kg? The required dose of dopamine is to be diluted to 50 mL with sodium chloride 0.9%.

□ 1   27 mg of dopamine is needed for the initial dilution
□ 2   once diluted, a rate of 0.1 mL/hour provides a dose of 2.7 mcg/minute
□ 3   if a concentrated solution is needed the required dose of dopamine can be diluted to a volume of 8.5 mL with sodium chloride 0.9%

4   Child A is to receive meropenem as an intravenous infusion for *E. coli* sepsis resistant to other standard agents. Which of the following doses is/are suitable given that Child A is 2 years old, weighs 11 kg, and has an eGFR of 30 mL/minute/1.73m^2?

□ 1   110 mg every 12 hours
□ 2   220 mg every 12 hours
□ 3   110 mg every 8 hours

5   Which of the following is/are true regarding the correct quantity of drug to supply for the detailed patients?

□ 1   1 original pack of amoxicillin 125 mg/5mL suspension in a 3-year-old child who is to take '2.5 mL THREE times daily for 7 days' for a respiratory tract infection
□ 2   35 aciclovir 800 mg tablets to a 13-year-old boy being treated for chickenpox
□ 3   28 *Rifinah* 300 mg capsules for a 15-year-old boy being treated for 14 days at the maximum dose for pruritus due to cholestasis

6   You are asked to prepare a dopamine infusion for a man weighing 80 kg. He has been prescribed an infusion of 3 mcg/kg/minute. You have 5 mL ampoules at a concentration of 160 mg/mL available to you, which you are asked to dilute to a concentration of 1.6 mg/mL using sodium chloride 0.9%. Which of the following statements is/are correct?

□ 1   Each ampoule should be diluted to 400 mL
□ 2   In 1 hour the patient should receive 1.44 mg of dopamine
□ 3   The infusion rate should be set at 0.15 mL/minute.

7   A child weighing 25 kg is travelling to Uganda for 7 days. The child is
     of normal weight for their age. Which of the following options would
     be a suitable option for preventing malaria in this child?

     ☐ **1**   Doxycycline 100 mg capsules ×37
     ☐ **2**   *Lariam* 250 mg tablets ×6
     ☐ **3**   *Malarone* paediatric tablets ×30

CLASSIFICATION QUESTIONS

Amar Iqbal, Alistair Murray and Ryan Hamilton

> In this section, for each numbered question, select the one lettered option that most closely corresponds to the answer. Within each group of questions each lettered option may be used once, more than once, or not at all.

Questions 1–3 concern the following quantities:

A   50 g
B   100 g
C   150 g
D   200 g
E   250 g

1   The amount of white soft paraffin in a 500 g tub of '50:50 ointment' that you have just supplied on a FP10 prescription to a 16-year-old for use as an emollient for eczema
2   A suitable amount of *E45* cream to be applied twice daily to both hands of a 12-year-old child for a period of 2 weeks to help relieve contact dermatitis
3   The amount of liquid paraffin in 500 g of *Epaderm* ointment, which is to be used as a soap substitute in a 5-year-old child who has presented to hospital with signs suggestive of atopic eczema

Questions 4 and 5 concern the following dose volumes:

A   1.5 mL
B   2.5 mL
C   5 mL
D   7 mL
E   9 mL

4   The dose volume of co-amoxiclav 125/315 mL suspension for a 5-year-old child weighing 20 kg who has severe renal impairment (eGFR = 15 mL/minute/1.73m^2)

5   The maximum dose volume of itraconazole 10 mg/mL suspension in a 5-year-old child of average weight being treated for pityriasis versicolor

Questions 6 and 7 concern the following quantities of sodium chloride, which are to be added to water to make an aqueous solution:

A   0.09 g
B   0.45 g
C   0.9 g
D   4.5 g
E   9.0 g

6   60 mL of a 1.5% solution
7   45 mL of a solution which, when diluted with an equal volume of water, results in a 10% solution

For questions 8–10, please choose the ONE answer from the list below that is correct.

A   240 units
B   2400 units
C   24 000 units
D   224 000 units
E   240 000 units

8   How many units of protease does a patient receive over 4 weeks if they are taking 5 × *Creon* 40 000 capsules daily?
9   How many units of insulin are in 2.4 L of *Lantus* injection?
10   How many units of colecalciferol are contained in 60 × *Adcal-D3* tablets?

For questions 11 and 12, please choose the ONE answer from the list below that is correct.

A   1.5 kg
B   3 kg
C   4.5 kg
D   6 kg
E   7.5 kg

11   How much emulsifying wax should be used to make 15 kg of Emulsifying Ointment BP?

12 How much white soft paraffin is used to make 6 kg of Emulsifying Ointment BP?

For questions 13 and 14, consider the following:

A syringe driver is set up containing 360 mg diamorphine in 20 mL of 0.9% sodium chloride solution to be given over 24 hours. What volume of diamorphine solution will the patient have received after the following lengths of time, to the nearest 0.1 mL? Choose ONE answer for each question from the list below:
    A   3.3 mL
    B   3.7 mL
    C   4.5 mL
    D   6.0 mL
    E   6.6 mL

13 4 hours and 27 minutes
14 7 hours and 58 minutes

Questions 15–18 concern the following regular doses of paracetamol:
    A   50 mg every 12 hours
    B   200 mg every 8 hours
    C   500 mg every 6 to 8 hours
    D   500 mg every 4 to 6 hours
    E   1 g every 4 to 6 hours

You are a paediatric specialist pharmacist undertaking a ward visit on the children's wards. During your visits you need to calculate doses of paracetamol for your patients.
Which doses from the list above are most appropriate for the following patients?

15 An 8-year-old boy weighing 26 kg requiring oral paracetamol for post-operative pain after removal of his appendix.
16 A 9-year-old receiving regular haemodialysis and weighing 34 kg who requires intravenous paracetamol for pain and discomfort.
17 A 1-week-old baby born after 27 weeks' gestation requiring oral para-cetamol for pyrexia.
18 A 10-year-old girl requiring paracetamol suspension for postoperative pain.

STATEMENT QUESTIONS

Amar Iqbal and Alistair Murray

> The questions in this section consist of a statement in the top row followed by a second statement beneath.
>
> You need to:
>
> decide whether the *first statement* is true or false
>
> decide whether the *second statement* is true or false
>
> Then choose:
>
> A   if both statements are true and the second statement is *a correct explanation* of the first statement
>
> B   if both statements are true but the second statement is *not a correct explanation* of the first statement
>
> C   if the first statement is true but the second statement is false
>
> D   if the first statement is false but the second statement is true
>
> E   if both statements are false

1   You are asked to review a prescription for a continuous subcutaneous maintenance infusion pump of apomorphine 20 mg, which is due to be prescribed for Mr ST who has severe Parkinson's disease. The pump is to run for 12 hours each day and Mr ST weighs 60 kg.

First statement

The pump should be set at a rate of approximately 1.7 mg/hour

Second statement

The usual maintenance rate is 15–60 mcg/kg/hour

2   The dietician on your ward has recommended *Nutrini® Multi Fibre Liquid* for a 2-year-old child on the paediatric ward for disease-related malnutrition.

First statement

Nutrini® Multi Fibre Liquid contains 100 kcal of energy per bottle

Second statement

1 kcal of energy is equivalent to approximately 4.2 kJ

3   Child R who is 32 weeks' gestational age and weighs 2 kg has been recommended some arginine as an intravenous infusion over 12 hours as his metabolic results suggests he has high levels of ammonia due to a citrullinaemia.

First statement

Child R will receive approximately 863 mg of arginine over the course of the infusion

Second statement

Arginine is given at an initial dose of 300 mg/kg over 90 minutes, followed by 12.5 mg/kg/hour

4   The paediatric ward nurse asks for you to double-check her syringe pump calculation for daily fluid requirement in Child F, who is 3 years old and weighs 15 kg.

First statement

A bag of sodium chloride 0.9% and glucose 10% run at a rate of 52 mL/hour will provide adequate fluid replacement

Second statement

Child F needs 1250 mL of fluid replacement per day

5   There is a supply problem with sodium bicarbonate 4.2% intravenous infusion. The resuscitation team ask for your advice on how to dilute the 8.4% infusion so that they can provide this information to their team members.

First statement

A 1:1 dilution of the 8.4% sodium bicarbonate solution will give a 4.2% solution

Second statement

An equal volume of each product is required to provide a solution that is half the strength of the original

6 **First statement**

The maximum rate of a dose of vancomycin given intravenously to a 3-week-old neonate born at 28 weeks' gestation weighing 2 kg for a Gram-positive bacterial soft-tissue infection would be 0.5 mg/minute

Second statement

The correct dose for a child of this age is 30 mg, which should be given over at least 60 minutes

7 For an adult with moderate acute asthma:

First statement

The maximum recommended dose of salbutamol via a nebuliser is 10 mg in 1 hour

Second statement

The maximum recommended dose of salbutamol from a metered dose inhaler used with a large volume spacer during 1 hour is 6 mg

Open book answers

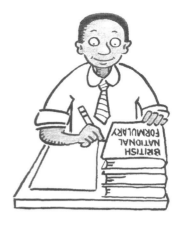

SIMPLE COMPLETION ANSWERS

1 C
See BNF, Chapter 5 (Infections), section 5.1, Antibacterial drugs, Choice of a suitable drug, which mentions all the listed options except the need to consider formulation

2 C
See BNFC, Chapter 9 (Nutrition and blood), section 9.8.2. Acute porphyria attacks are uncommon before puberty

3 C
Flucloxacillin is a safe option and useful in staphylococcal skin infections. The other agents are either unsafe in acute porphyria or unsuitable for the given condition

4 E
See BNF, Chapter 5 (Infections), section 5.1.4. Gentamicin can be used for the following intravenous indications: septicaemia, neonatal sepsis, meningitis and other CNS infections, biliary-tract infection, acute pyelonephritis or prostatitis, endocarditis and pneumonia (hospital patients only), and it is used as an adjunct in listerial meningitis. It is not indicated for urinary-tract infections

5 D
Ototoxicity is an irreversible side-effect of gentamicin

6 C
See BNF, Chapter 2 (Cardiovascular system), section 2.12. Simvastatin is given at a maximum dose of 20 mg daily with concomitant amiodarone, verapamil, diltiazem, amlodipine, or ranolazine

7 C
See BNF, Chapter 2 (Cardiovascular system), section 2.12. Statins can cause myopathy (muscle pain, tenderness, and weakness) and rarely interstitial lung disease (dyspnoea, cough, and weight loss). Patients must seek medical attention immediately if they experience these symptoms

8 E
See BNF, Chapter 2 (Cardiovascular system), section 2.12. Thyroid function tests are necessary in order to rule out hypothyroidism. Correcting hypothyroidism may resolve any lipid abnormality

9 C
See BNF, Chapter 10 (Musculoskeletal and joint diseases), section 10.1.3. Methotrexate does not need to be used with caution in those with a raised neutrophil count; however, it must be stopped immediately if there is a clinically significant drop in neutrophil count

10 E
See BNF, Chapter 10 (Musculoskeletal and joint diseases), section 10.1.3. Methotrexate requires routine monitoring of full blood count, renal and liver function tests

11 E
See BNF, Chapter 10 (Musculoskeletal and joint diseases), section 10.1.3. Methotrexate is not known to precipitate diabetes

12 B
See BNF, Chapter 10 (Musculoskeletal and joint diseases), section 10.1.3. Co-codamol is the safest analgesic to purchase over-the-counter while on methotrexate. Use of aspirin or NSAIDs will necessitate careful monitoring, hence they are not recommended

13 E
See BNF, Chapter 13 (Skin), section 13.10.4. The manufacturer recommends 2 × 30 g packs for adequate treatment. However, the table entitled 'Suitable quantities of parascitidal preparations' suggests 30–60 g for a single application. Thus, 60–120 g is needed for two applications (NB: 120 g is the maximum recommended quantity)

14 E
See BNF, Chapter 13 (Skin), section 13.10.4. The manufacturer recommends that the product should not be applied to the head and neck

15 A
See BNF, Chapter 14 (Immunological products and vaccines), section 14.1. Individuals with a previous history of anaphylactic reactions to egg should not be given tick-borne encephalitis vaccine and yellow fever vaccine. Influenza vaccines may be given but such individuals should be referred to a specialist in hospital in order to have the vaccine, with facilities available to treat anaphylaxis

16 E
See BNF, Chapter 14 (Immunological products and vaccines), section 14.4. Typhoid oral vaccine is given on days 1, 3 and 5. It takes 7–10 days to confer protection following the last dose

17 E
See BNF, Chapter 14 (Immunological products and vaccines), section 14.1. Contraindications to MMR include: immunosuppression; those who have received another live vaccine by injection within 4 weeks; those who have had an anaphylactic reaction to excipients such as gelatin and neomycin; if given to women, pregnancy should be avoided for 1 month

18 D
See BNF, Chapter 6 (Endocrine system), section 6.4.1.1. A preparation containing oestrogen and preogestogen is recommended for women with an intact uterus

19 C
See BNF, Chapter 7 (Obstetrics, gynaecology, and urinary-tract disorders), section 7.3. Hormonal contraception is the most effective method of contraception, whereas intrauterine devices are a highly effective alternative form of contraception. Barrier methods are less effective but reliable

20 E
Paracetamol is the safest analgesic in pregnancy

21 B
See BNF, Chapter 2 (Cardiovascular system), section 2.5.5.1. Captopril, enalapril, and quinapril should be avoided in the first few weeks following delivery, especially in preterm infants, due to the risk of neonatal hypotension

22 E
The endorsement 'SLS' should be on the prescription (see Drug Tariff Part VIIIA for more information on the reasoning for this)

23 D
See BNF, Chapter 4 (Central nervous system), section 4.7.1. See individual drug monograph for the symbol denoting that this product is less suitable for prescribing

24 B
There is one formulation of the same drug prescribed; this attracts a single NHS levy

25 E
Cilest contains the active ingredients in two different pills (this carries two charges).Both mefenamic acid and tranexamic acid carry a single charge each. A total of four charges apply

26 D
See BNF, Chapter 9 (Nutrition and blood), section 9.1.5. Nitrofurantoin carries a definite risk of haemolysis

27 C
See BNFC, General reference section for a list of E numbers

28 C
See BNF, Chapter 4 (Central nervous system), section 4.2.1 See table entitled 'Equivalent doses of oral antipsychotics'. 100 mg chlorpromazine is equivalent to 50 mg clozapine

29 B
See BNF, Chapter 2 (Cardiovascular system), section 2.4. Diabetes is not listed as a cautioned use for beta-blockers; however, do note that beta-blockers can mask the symptoms of hypoglycaemia

30 B
See BNF, Chapter 2 (Cardiovascular system), section 2.3.2. An echocardiogram is not needed when initiating amiodarone

31 C
See BNF, Chapter 6 (Endocrine system), section 6.3.2. See table entitled 'Equivalent anti-inflammatory doses of corticosteroids'. A 5 mg dose of prednisolone is equivalent to 20 mg of hydrocortisone

32 E
Where an ACEI is causing persistent or troublesome coughing, the alternative product is an ARB (angiotensin II receptor blocker).

33 E
See BNF, Chapter 13 (Skin), section 13.4. *Synalar* 1 in 10 dilution is a mild corticosteroid.

34 D
See BNF, Chapter 13 (Skin), section 13.4. See table entitled 'Suitable quantities of corticosteroid preparations to be prescribed for specific areas of the body'. When used as a single application, both legs require 100 g for 2 weeks, and the trunk requires 100 g. This is equivalent to two tubes for single application; in this case it is a twice-daily application, hence 4 tubes are needed

35 A
See BNF, Chapter 7 (Obstetrics, gynaecology, and urinary-tract disorders), section 7.3. Reasons to stop immediately include sudden chest pain, sudden breathlessness (or cough with blood-stained sputum), unexplained swelling or pain in calf of one leg, severe stomach pain, serious neurological effects (e.g. prolonged first presentation of a headache, sudden loss of vision, sudden loss of hearing, syncope, dysphasia, marked numbness affecting one side of the body, and unexplained first seizure), liver-related problems (e.g. hepatitis, jaundice, and hepatomegaly), raised blood pressure (above systolic 160 mmHg or diastolic 95 mmHg), prolonged immobility following leg injury or surgery, and detection of any risk factor which contraindicates treatment

36 C
See BNF, Chapter 9 (Nutrition and blood), section 9.3 – *Kabiven* contains 4 mmol/L of magnesium ions

37 D
See BNF, Chapter 2 (Cardiovascular system), section 2.3.2. Signs of breathlessness may indicate pulmonary toxicity (usually seen as pneumonitis and fibrosis) and will necessitate a review of the drug

38 D
For BNF Guidance on Prescribing in palliative care, see table entitled 'Equivalent doses of morphine sulfate and diamorphine given over 24 hours'. As a general rule the daily dose of diamorphine is $^1/_3$ the total daily oral morphine dose

39 B
See BNF, Chapter 9 (Nutrition and blood), section 9.1.1. See table entitled 'Iron content of different iron salts'. Ferrous sulfate contains 60 mg of ferrous iron per tablet and *Fersamal* contains 45 mg of ferrous iron per 5 mL spoonful. Giving a 10 mL b.d. dose of *Fersamal* provides 180 mg of ferrous iron (which is the same as taking ferrous sulfate 200 mg TDS)

40 C
See BNF Appendix 4, Intravenous additives

41 C
See BNF, Chapter 4 (Central nervous system), section 4.3.2. A 3-week interval is needed before starting phenelzine following discontinuation of clomipramine or imipramine. For all other antidepressants, a 2-week interval is needed before starting an MAOI (or 1–2 weeks if a TCA or related drug)

42 E
Topical erythromycin has little potential for interaction with prednisolone. Options A and C have the potential to affect absorption profiles of the interacting drugs. Option B is a significant interaction. Option D carries a caution related to prolongation of QT intervals, hence affecting cardiac rhythm

43 E
Patches should be folded upon themselves once the backing paper has been removed and then disposed of accordingly

44 D
Using the BNF Appendix 'Cardiovascular Risk Prediction Charts' for primary prevention, it can be seen that Mr FZ has a >20% risk over the next 10 years based on his high blood pressure and TC:HDL ratio

45 E
See BNF, Chapter 4 (Central nervous system), section 4.7.4.1. *Zomig* is the brand name for zolmitriptan

46 A
See BNF, Chapter 5 (Infections), section 5.3.5. See drug monograph for dosing

47 B
See BNF, Chapter 13 (Skin), section 13.4. Clobetasone butyrate (*Eumovate*) can be sold to the public in pack sizes of 15 g or less for short-term symptomatic treatment of eczema and dermatitis (but not seborrhoeic dermatitis) in adults and children over 12 years of age

48 C
See BNF, Chapter 3 (Respiratory system), section 3.4.3 for the adrenaline monograph or Appendix entitled 'Medical emergencies in the community'

49 B
See BNF, Chapter 6 (Endocrine system), section 6.2.2 or a good OTC reference book. Any non-specific illness to carbimazole must be immediately referred to a medical professional to rule out bone marrow suppression (such as neutropenia and agranulocytosis)

50 A
See BNF, Chapter 8 (Malignant disease and immunosuppression), section 8.1.3. Cytarabine exists as a lipid formulation for intrathecal use. Vinca alkaloids (such as options C, D, and E) are for intravenous use only as intrathecal use can cause severe neurotoxicity, which is usually fatal

MULTIPLE COMPLETION ANSWERS

1 C
See BNF Chapter 5 (Infections); section 5.3.2.2.
Only ganciclovir and foscarnet are active against CMV infections. Aciclovir is not clinically useful because CMV is relatively resistant to aciclovir

2 A
See BNF, Chapter 9 (Nutrition and blood); section 9.1.1.2.
According to the BNF iron may be administered parenterally as iron isomaltoside 1000, ferumoxytol, iron sucrose. Parenteral iron is generally reserved for use when oral therapy is unsuccessful

3 C
See BNF, Chapter 8 (Malignant disease and immunosuppression); section 8.1, Cytotoxic drugs, Side-effects of cytoxic drugs, nausea and vomiting. Drugs may be divided according to their 'emetogenic' potential, but the symptoms vary according to the dose, to other drugs administered, and to individual susceptibility. Patients vary in their susceptibility to drug-induced nausea and vomiting; those affected more often include women, patients under 50 years of age, anxious patients, and those who experience motion sickness. Susceptibility also increases with repeated exposure to the cytotoxic drug

4 A
See BNF, individual drug monographs. Seizure is a possible side-effect of all the medicines listed, thus in a high-risk patient, the risk of seizure is higher and the patient must be closely monitored

5 E
See BNF, Chapter 7 (Obstetrics, gynaecology, and urinary-tract disorders); section 7.3.5.
No prescription is needed to purchase the morning after pill i.e. levonorgestrel (*Levonelle*). It is most effective within 12 hours but can be taken up to 72 hours after coitus. However, it is contraindicated in patients with acute porphyria

6 A
See BNFC, General Guidance

ANSWERS

7 D
See MEP 38, section 3.4, Wholesale Dealing. Any person acting as a wholesale distributor has to hold a wholesale distribution authorisation, therefore not all healthcare professionals can receive medications by wholesale. The MHRA and the European Commission provide that distributors and persons trading in medicines must comply with the principles of and guidelines for Good Distribution Practice

8 A
See MEP 38, section 3.6, Veterinary Medicines.
   Identification of the animal, withdrawal period (if there is one), and the words for 'animal treatment only' are all required on a label when a product is supplied 'for use under the cascade'

9 A
See BNF Guidance on Prescribing in palliative care; Syringe drivers

10 D
The medical term for kidney stones is renal calculus. See Topiramate, side-effects

11 B

12 B
See BNF, Chapter 6 (Endocrine system).
   Hormone replacement therapy (HRT) is given to women to alleviate menopausal symptoms. Women with an intact uterus should receive an oestrogen as well as a progesterone. Women without a uterus would be prescribed an oestrogen only

13 A
See BNF, Appendix 5 (Breastfeeding).

14 E
See BNF, Appendix 2 (Liver disease).

15 B
See BNF, Chapter 14 (Immunological products and vaccines), section 14.1, Immunisation schedule. Diphtheria and pneumococcal polysaccharide conjugate vaccine are given at 2 months along with the first dose of the rotavirus vaccine. Meningococcal group C conjugate vaccine is given at 3 months

16 A

17 B
See BNF, Emergency treatment of poisoning. Barbiturates and phenothiazines are associated with hypothermia in patients who overdose, whereas hyperthermia is associated with drugs that have antimuscarinic properties such as diphenhydramine

18 B
See MEP 38, Patient Group Directives

19 A
See BNF, Chapter 4, (Central nervous system), section 4.7.2. Long-term use of opioid analgesics can cause hypogonadism and adrenal insufficiency in both men and women. This is thought to be dose-related and can lead to amenorrhoea, reduced libido, infertility, depression, and erectile dysfunction. Long-term use of opioid analgesics has also been associated with a state of abnormal pain sensitivity (hyperalgesia). Pain associated with hyperalgesia is usually distinct from pain associated with disease progression or breakthrough pain, and is often more diffuse and less defined

20 C
See BNF, Chapter 4 (Central nervous system), section 4.2.1. Aripiprazole is associated with a low risk of weight gain, whereas olanzapine has a high risk of causing weight gain, and clozapine also commonly causes weight gain

ANSWERS

21 E
See BNF Chapter 2 (Cardiovascular system), section 2.1.1, Digoxin, cautions.
  Hypercalcaemia can increase risk of digitalis toxicity because calcium ions act synergistically with digitalis and may cause toxic arrhythmias, cardiac arrest and may be fatal. High levels of potassium (hyperkalaemia) and magnesium (hypermagnesaemia) seem to help prevent digitalis toxicity

22 A
See BNF, Chapter 6 (Endocrine system), section 6.3.2. The CSM has recommended that gradual withdrawal of systemic corticosteroids should be considered in those where disease is unlikely to relapse and who have:

1   recently received repeated courses
2   taken a short course within 1 year of stopping long-term therapy
3   other possible causes of adrenal suppression
4   received more than 40 mg daily of prednisolone
5   been given repeat doses in the evening
6   received more than three weeks' treatment

23 C
See BNF, Chapter 10 (Musculoskeletal and joint diseases), section 10.1.3. Leflunomide requires washout procedure before starting another DMARD. Either colestyramine or the use of charcoal would be appropriate for the washout procedure.

24 A
See BNF, Chapter 8 (Malignant disease and immunosuppression), section 8.1, Anthracycline, side-effects.
  Dexrazoxane, an iron chelator, is licensed for the prevention of chronic cumulative cardiotoxicity caused by doxorubicin or epirubicin treatment in advanced or metastatic breast cancer patients who have received a prior cumulative dose of 300 mg/m^2 of doxorubicin or a prior cumulative dose of 540 mg/m^2 of epirubicin when further anthracycline treatment is required. Patients receiving dexrazoxane should still be monitored for cardiac toxicity

25 A
Latin abbreviations are found in the the BNF

26 A
See BNF, Chapter 6 (Endocrine system), section 6.6.2.
   Strontium ranelate stimulates bone formation and reduces bone resorption. Strontium ranelate is contraindicated in patients who suffer from a current or previous venous thromboembolic event (ischaemic heart disease, peripheral arterial disease, or cerebrovascular disease), uncontrolled hypertension, or temporary or prolonged immobilisation. Strontium ranelate treatment has been associated with an increased risk of serious cardiovascular disease, including myocardial infarction, and the risk should be assessed before treatment and regularly during treatment. Strontium ranelate should be initiated only by specialists for the treatment of severe postmenopausal osteoporosis in women at high-risk of fracture, or for severe osteoporosis in men at increased risk of fracture.

27 B
See BNF, Chapter 6 (Endocrine system), section 6.4.1.1. Patients with epilepsy should use HRT with caution; however, liver disease and DVT is contraindicated

28 B
During the first 2 weeks after fertilisation, teratogens have almost no effect on the fetus. However, if the pregnant woman is exposed to high doses of teratogenic substance it can destroy the embryo. Any exposure after this initial period may cause fetal abnormalities, either structural or behavioural

29 A
See BNF, Appendix 1 (Interactions)

30 B
See BNF, Chapter 6 (Endocrine system), section 6.1.2.1. The use of sulfonylureas in pregnancy should generally be avoided because of the risk of neonatal hypoglycaemia

31 A
See BNF, Appendix 1 (Interactions)

ANSWERS

32 A
See BNF, Chapter 6 (Endocrine system), section 6.1.6. Self-monitoring of blood-glucose concentration is appropriate for patients with type 2 'diabetes': who are treated with insulin; who are treated with oral hypoglycaemic drugs, e.g. sulfonylureas, to provide information on hypoglycaemia; to monitor changes in blood-glucose concentration resulting from changes in lifestyle or medication, and during intercurrent illness; to ensure safe blood-glucose concentration during activities, including driving

33 B
Enalapril has no effect on QT interval. However, many other classes of drugs such as tricyclic antidepressants do prolong QT interval, and should be used with caution in patients with arrhythmias

34 B
Fosamax tablets should be swallowed whole with plenty of water while sitting or standing. This is due to severe oesophageal reactions having been reported. The tablet should be taken on an empty stomach at least 30 minutes before breakfast and the patient should stand or sit upright for at least 30 minutes after taking the tablet

35 A
See BNF, Chapter 7 (Obstetrics, gynaecology and urinary-tract disorders), section 7.1.1.

36 C
See BNF, Chapter 6 (Endocrine system), section 6.3.2. Mineralocorticoid side-effects are associated with hypertension, sodium and water retention, and potassium and calcium loss

37 A
See BNF, Chapter 9 (Nutrition and blood), section 9.1.5.

38 D
See BNF, Chapter 8 (Malignant disease and immunosuppression), section 8.1. Bleomycin and vincristine are the only cytotoxics that do not cause bone marrow depression

39 C
Bumetanide causes hyponatraemia as a side-effect. Fluoxetine is a selective serotonin reuptake inhibitor (SSRI). The CSM has advised that hyponatraemia has been associated with all types of antidepressants; however, it has been reported more frequently with SSRIs

40 A
See BNF, Appendix 3, Renal impairment

41 D
See MEP 38, Patient Group Directives

42 B
See BNFC, Chapter 11 (Eye), section 11.3.1

43 A
See BNF, Chapter 10 (Musculoskeletal and joint diseases). Diuretics reduce urate excretion by both directly and indirectly increasing urate reabsorption and decreasing urate secretion. Aspirin also increases the level of uric acid

44 A
See BNFC, Chapter 14 (Active immunity), section 14.4, side-effects: 'The vaccine should not be withheld from children with a history to a preceding dose of: fever, irrespective of severity; persistent crying or screaming for more than 3 hours; severe local reaction, irrespective of extent.'

45 A
See BNFC, Chapter 13 (Skin), section 13.4

46 A
See BNFC, Chapter 6 (Endocrine system), section 6.2.1. Hypothyroidism is also known as juvenile myxoedema, and lymphadenoid goitre is known as Hashimoto's thyroiditis

47 B
See MEP 38, Destruction of controlled drugs

ANSWERS

48 B
See BNF, Chapter 4 (Central nervous system), section 4.1. Addition of beta-blockers, antidepressants, and antipsychotics should be **avoided** where possible. Counselling can be of considerable help both during and after the taper

49 D
See BNF, Chapter 7 (Obstetrics, gynaecology and urinary-tract disorders).

Microgynon is a combined oral contraceptive. The critical time for loss of contraceptive protection is when a pill is omitted at the beginning or end of a cycle. If a woman forgets to take a pill, it should be taken as soon as she remembers and the next one taken at the normal time. If the delay is 24 hours or longer, she should continue taking the pill normally. Consequently, she will not be protected for the next 7 days and must use alternative methods of contraception. If these 7 days run beyond the end of the packet, the next packet should be started. *Microgynon* does not have any inactive tablets. It is a 21-day cycle pill, and therefore the patient should omit the pill-free interval

50 E
Cardiac troponins T and I are the preferred markers for myocardial injury as they have the highest sensitivities and specificities for the diagnosis of acute myocardial infarction. There will also be increased levels of C-reactive protein (CRP) and creatine kinase (CK-MB) following a myocardial infarction event

CLASSIFICATION ANSWERS

1 D
See BNF

2 B

3 A

4 E

5 E
See BNF, Appendix 1 (potentially serious interactions are marked with a black dot)

6 B

7 C

8 A

9 A
See BNF, Chapter 11 (Eye), section 11.8.2

10 C
See BNF, Chapter 9 (Nutrition and blood), section 9.1.3

11 E
See BNF, Chapter 4 (Central nervous system), section 4.7.2

12 D
See BNF, Chapter 9 (Nutrition and blood), section 9.1.2

13 D
See BNF, Appendix 3. Erythromycin tablets are enteric coated

14 A

15 B

16 E
See BNF, Appendix 3. Absorption of doxycycline is not significantly affected by milk as with many other tetracyclines

17 C
See BNF, Chapter 7 (Obstetrics, gynaecology, and urinary-tract disorders), section 7.1.3. Beta$_2$ agonists can be used to inhibit uncomplicated premature labour between 24 and 33 weeks of gestation

18 D
See BNF, Chapter 6 (Endocrine system), section 6.1.4

19 A
See BNF, Chapter 9 (Nutrition and blood), section 9.1.5

20 B
See BNF, Chapter 6 (Endocrine system), section 6.1.2.2

21 A
See BNF, Chapter 3 (Respiratory system), section 3.4.3

22 D
See BNF, Chapter 4 (Central nervous system), section 4.3.1, contraindications

23 D
See BNF, Chapter 4 (Central nervous system), section 4.3.1, side-effects, endocrine effects

24 E
See BNF, Chapter 8 (Malignant disease and immunosuppression), section 8.3.4

25 E

26 C
One charge per item of hosiery

27 B

28 B
If the carbamazepine were prescribed for epilepsy, she could be entitled to a medical exemption certificate; this is not the case for other indications

29 C

30 E

31 C

32 D

33 D

34 A

35 C

36 B

37 E
See BNF, Chapter 9 (Nutrition and blood), section 9.2.2.1

38 A
See BNF, Chapter 9 (Nutrition and blood), section 9.1.2, folic acid, indications

39 D
See BNF, Chapter 2 (Cardiovascular system), section 2.3.2

40 B
See BNF, Chapter 5 (Infections), section 5.1.9

41 C

42 E

43 A

44 B

ANSWERS

45 D

46 E

47 A

48 D

49 C

50 B

STATEMENT ANSWERS

1 A
See BNF, Chapter 1 (Gastro-intestinal system), section 1.1.2. *Gastrocote* tablets have a high sugar content, and therefore should be used with caution in patients with diabetes

2 A
See BNF, Chapter 1 (Gastro-intestinal system), section 1.3.1. All H_2-receptor antagonists heal gastric and duodenal ulcers by reducing gastric acid output as a result of histamine H_2-receptor blockade

3 C
See BNF, Chapter 2 (Cardiovascular system), section 2.6.3. Ivabradine lowers the heart rate by its action on the sinus node

4 B
See BNF, Chapter 4 (Central nervous system), section 4.2.1 and NICE Guidance 178. All antipsychotic drugs should be considered on a patient-by-patient basis.
　　See BNF, Chapter 4 (Central nervous system), section 4.2.1. The CSM has advised that olanzapine is associated with an increased risk of stroke in elderly patients with dementia

5 C
See BNF, Chapter 4 (Central nervous system), section 4.6. Nausea in the first trimester of pregnancy is usually mild and does not require drug therapy. On rare occasions, if vomiting is severe, short-term treatment with an antihistamine such as promethazine may be required. Metoclopramide may be considered as second-line treatment

6 C
See BNF, Chapter 4 (Central nervous system), section 4.7.2. Pethidine should be avoided for the treatment of pain in patients with sickle-cell disease. This is due to accumulation of a neurotoxic metabolite, which can precipitate seizures

7 A
See BNF, Chapter 8 (Malignant disease and immunosuppression), section 8.2.2. Patients on ciclosporin therapy may develop hyperkalaemia. Patients' potassium levels should be monitored periodically during therapy

8 E
Low-sodium antacid preparations are a suitable choice for patients with hypertension.
See BNF, Chapter 1 (Gastro-intestinal system), section 1.1.2. *Peptac* liquid is not a low-sodium preparation, so is therefore not suitable for such patients

9 A
See BNF, Chapter 6 (Endocrine system), section 6.7.1. Dopaminergics can cause sudden onset of sleep and patients should exercise caution if driving. See notes on driving.

10 D
See BNF, Chapter 7 (Obstetrics, gynaecology, and urinary-tract disorders), section 7.1.2. Mifepristone is used for the termination of pregnancy. It acts by sensitising the myometrium to prostaglandin-induced contractions and ripens the cervix

11 B
See BNF, Chapter 6 (Endocrine system), section 6.1.3. Intravenous replacement of fluid and electrolytes with sodium chloride in isotonic solution given intravenously is an essential part of the management of ketoacidosis

12 E
See BNF, Chapter 9 (Nutrition and blood), section 9.6.3. Deficiency of vitamin C may cause scurvy. Vitamin C is a water-soluble vitamin

13 C
See BNF, Chapter 9 (Nutrition and blood), section 9.8.1. Penicillamine is used in Wilson's disease to help in the elimination of copper ions

14 B
See BNF, Chapter 4 (Central nervous system), section 4.3.1. Tricyclic antidepressants have anticholinergic side-effects.

See BNF, Chapter 12 (Ear, nose, and oropharynx), section 12.3.5. Artificial saliva can be of benefit in patients with dry mouth

15 A
See BNF, Chapter 10 (Musculoskeletal and joint diseases), section 10.1.3. Methotrexate may induce agranulocytosis. See notes on monitoring

16 A
See BNF, Appendix 1. St John's wort is a CYP450 inducer and causes the metabolism of darunavir to be increased

17 E
See BNF, Chapter 5 (Infections), section 5.3.2.2. Ganciclovir crosses the placenta and is potentially teratogenic, and therefore should be avoided in pregnancy

18 A
See BNF, Chapter 9 (Nutrition and blood), section 9.1.3. *Eprex* is epoetin alpha and is used to treat anaemia in renal failure, which is caused by insufficient erythropoietin production

19 A
See BNFC, Chapter 13 (Skin), section 13.2.1. Soap should be avoided in dry skin conditions.

See MHRA for the drug safety update on aqueous cream

20 C
See BNF, Chapter 13 (Skin), section 13.4. Hydrocortisone is a mild corticosteroid and supplying 15–30 g should be enough for use on the face

21 D
See BNF, Chapter 4 (Central nervous system), section 4.7.1. For patients weighing less than 50 kg, the IV dose should be calculated at 15 mg/kg. This can still be administered up to four times a day (4–6 hourly)

ANSWERS

22 E
See BNF, Chapter 2 (Cardiovascular system), section 2.12, simvastatin, dosing regimens
   See BNF, Appendix 1. Increased risk of myopathy due to increased serum concentrations of simvastatin

23 B
See BNF, Chapter 8 (Malignant disease and immunosuppression), section 8.1.4. Intrathecal administration of vinca alkaloids is usually fatal. Vincristine can cause neurotoxicity that may limit the acceptability of treatment

24 C
See BNF, Chapter 5 (Infections), section 5.1.2.1. Cross-over hypersensitivity caused by the beta-lactam ring in the structure of both drug classes

25 D
See BNF, Chapter 14 (Immunological products and vaccines), section 14.1, Active immunity, vaccines and HIV infection. The patient is not significantly immunocompromised and so may receive the varicella-zoster vaccine, which is a live-attenuated vaccine

26 C
See BNF, Chapter 14 (Immunological products and vaccines), section 14.1, Active immunity, vaccines and HIV infection. The patient is at risk of flu. An injection would be preferable in these patients as the virus is inactivated.

27 B
See BNF, Appendix 5. Alginate is suitable for adsorbing moderate and heavy amounts of exudate

28 B
You have a professional duty to discuss all options available to your patient. See MEP 38, section 3.5.13 and GPhC guidance for more information. Also see BNF, Chapter 4 (Central nervous system), section 4.10.2 for licensed nicotine replacement options

29 E
Professional decision making is needed – 'she may have taken about 20 mL' means you cannot be sure how much the child has received, and it is unlikely the parent can accurately state how much has been removed from the bottle. In these circumstances you would advise the parent to take their child to hospital

See BNFC, Emergency treatment of poisoning. Doses as low as 75 mg/kg given within 60 minutes may cause hepatotoxicity.

30 C
See BNFC, Chapter 3 (Respiratory system), section 3.1.5. Children under the age of 5 years old should receive a spacer. Spacers should be washed with detergent once a month, and not rinsed

31 A
See BNFC, Chapter 3 (Respiratory system), section 3.1, Management of acute asthma, moderate acute asthma.

British Thoracic Society (BTS) and Scottish Intercollegiate Guidance Network (SIGN) guidance on asthma states the use of beta agonists with a spacer is as effective as, and better tolerated than, a nebuliser in mild to moderate exacerbations of asthma

32 B
See BNFC, Chapter 14 (Immunological products and vaccines), section 14.4. The patient has asthma and so is in a high-risk group. Intranasal *Fluenz* is preferred for patients aged between 2–18 years as it affords better protection than the inactivated injections

33 B
See BNF, Chapter 2 (Cardiovascular system), section 2.8.2. Patients with an INR of 5.0–8.0 but with no bleeding should withhold one or two doses of warfarin and reduce the maintenance dose

34 A
See BNF, Chapter 2 (Cardiovascular system), section 2.8.2. Patients taking warfarin for atrial fibrillation should aim for an INR of 2.5 (acceptable INR is 0.5 units each way)

35 E
See GPhC guidance on confidentiality. You only need to disclose the specific information required

ANSWERS

36 D
See RPS guidance. Clinical audits are not meant to assess individual staff but to determine whether the service is being delivered to best practice standards

37 B
See RPS guidance. Audits are used to identify ways to make improvements, and this is a cyclical process followed by re-audits. Improvements are not suggested to allow for re-audits to occur

38 E
See GPhC standards for CPD. You need to meet 50% of the recording criteria. If your CPD is not of expected quality you will be given feedback and may be asked to undertake further CPD

39 A
See MEP 38, section 3.5.11. There is no robust evidence supporting the use of homeopathy

40 D
See MEP, section 3.5.15 and GPhC guidance. It is necessary to assess the competence of all patients

41 A
See BNFC, Chapter 9 (Nutrition and blood), section 9.6.7. *Abidec* contains arachis (peanut) oil

42 B
See RPS guidance on the sale and supply of sumatriptan without a prescription

43 B
See BNF, Chapter 6 (Endocrine system), section 6.1.1, Drugs used in diabetes, Insulins, renal impairment

44 C
See BNFC, Chapter 2 (Cardiovascular system), section 2.5.1.2. Sildenafil increases the vasodilatory effects of nitric oxide

45 C
See GPhC guidance on the provision of pharmacy services affected by religious and moral beliefs.

See BNF, Chapter 7 (Obstetrics, gynaecology, and urinary-tract disorders), section 7.3.5. You should refer/signpost this patient to somewhere that will supply EHC, which may not be the patient's GP. This is especially important in the case of levonogestrel, which is only licensed for use within 72 hours of unprotected intercourse

46 D
See BNF, Dental Practitioners' Formulary. Erythromycin capsules are not included in the formulary, so erythromycin tablets should be prescribed instead

47 E
See BNFC, Chapter 2 (Cardiovascular system), section 2.5.5.1. Suitable licensed liquid preparations are available, and therefore it is illegal to compound or make a special formulation

48 A
See BNF, Chapter 4 (Central nervous system), section 4.8.1. See also MHRA/CHM guidance. Phenytoin falls into category 1 of anticonvulsants, so patients should be maintained on a specific manufacturer's product

49 B
See BNF, Guidance on prescribing, Prescribing in palliative care, Continuous subcutaneous infusions. Certain drugs can be combined into the same syringe, but the decision to use a syringe driver is made with regard to the patient's condition

50 A
See BNF, Chapter 5 (Infections), section 5.1.13, Urinary-tract infections, Renal impairment. See also BNF, Chapter 5 (Infections), section 5.1.13, Urinary-tract infections, Nitrofurantoin

ANSWERS

Closed book answers

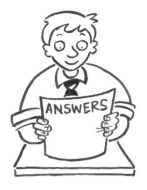

1 E
See BNF, Appendix 1. This patient should not receive trimethoprim because it is an antifolate and will interact with methotrexate

2 B
See BNF, Chapter 10 (Musculoskeletal and joint diseases), section 10.1.3. Folic acid should be given on any day that is different from the methotrexate dose

3 B
See BNF, Chapter 2 (Cardiovascular system), section 2.2.1. Thiazide diuretics can cause hyperglycaemia

4 C
See MEP 38 and GPhC CPD standards. You can submit your CPD by paper or mixed formats, as long as it complies with the standards for good CPD recording

5 B
See BNF, Chapter 10 (Musculoskeletal and joint diseases), section 10.1.1. Naproxen is an NSAID with a significant risk of gastrointestinal side-effects

6 B
See BNF, Appendix 1. Important interaction between clopidogrel with omeprazole and esomeprazole, leading to reduced effectiveness of clopidogrel

7 E
See MEP 38, section 3.3.10.2. Full packs can be supplied, thus a full calendar pack should be supplied

8 E
See BNF, Chapter 4 (Central nervous system), section 4.6, Drugs used in nausea and vertigo, Vomiting in pregnancy. This patient is in the first trimester, so her nausea should be self-limiting and drug treatment is not necessary

9 E
See BNF, Chapter 6 (Endocrine system), section 6.2.2, Antithyroid drugs, Neutropenia and agranulocytosis. This patient needs to be referred to her GP for further investigations

10 E
See MEP 38, section 3.2.5. Children under 6 years of age should be given simple cough syrups, or encouraged to drink plenty of fluids

11 C
See BNF, Chapter 3 (Respiratory system), section 3.4.1. Chlorphenamine is the only sedating antihistamine, which would not be suitable for a security guard

12 C
See BNF, Chapter 10 (Musculoskeletal and joint diseases), section 10.1.1. NSAIDs increase the risk of gastrointestinal bleeding, as does hepatic impairment and increased alcohol intake

13 A
See BNFC, Chapter 2 (Cardiovascular system), section 2.9. Aspirin associated with development of Reye's syndrome in children.
  See BNFC, Chapter 10 (Musculoskeletal and joint diseases), section 10.1.1. The other listed drugs may be used to treat postsurgical pain in children

14 E
See MEP 38, Appendix 6 and GPhC guidance on raising concerns. You should report concerns to your line manager, and/or the line manager of the pharmacist you have a concern about, before reporting it to the GPhC

15 C
See BNF, Chapter 2 (Cardiovascular system), section 2.1.1, Cardiac glycosides, Digoxin, side-effects

16 B
See BNF, Chapter 2 (Cardiovascular system), section 2.1.1. Hypokalaemia may precipitate digoxin toxicity

17 D
See BNF, Chapter 10 (Musculoskeletal and joint diseases), section 10.1.1. Pupil dilation is not a listed side-effect of NSAIDs

18 D
See NICE Clinical Guidance 91. Cognitive Behavioural Therapy, and similar individual or group therapies, are listed as first-line options for patients with newly diagnosed depression and a long-term condition

Week(s)	5 mg tablets	2.5 mg tablets
1 (20 mg)	4 × 7 = 28	--
2 (17.5 mg)	3 × 7 = 21	1 × 7 = 7
3 (15 mg)	3 × 7 = 21	--
4 (12.5 mg)	2 × 7 = 14	1 × 7 = 7
5 (10 mg)	2 × 7 = 14	--
6 (7.5 mg)	1 × 7 = 7	1 × 7 = 7
7 & 8 (5 mg)	1 × 14 = 14	--
9 & 10 (2.5 mg)	--	1 × 14 = 14
Total	119	35

ANSWERS

19 E
See MEP 38, section 3.6. Because this product is licensed for use in this disease in this species, it is not necessary to follow the veterinary prescribing cascade

Total volume (of double-strength peppermint water)	Volume of concentrated peppermint water	Volume of water
20 mL	1 mL	19 mL
100 mL	5 mL	95 mL
500 mL	25 mL	475 mL

20 B
See MEP 38, section 3.7.11. CD registers must be retained for at least 2 years after the last entry is made

21 A
See BNF, Appendix 3 and Chapter 2 (Cardiovascular system), section 2.3.2. Amiodarone can cause phototoxic reactions

22 B
See *British Pharmacopoeia*, Appendix XVIII. Filtration used when the methods of terminal sterilisation cannot be used

23 E
See MEP 38, section 2.9 and GPhC standards for CPD. Pharmacists are encouraged to use multiple, and varied methods to undertake CPD

24 D
See BNFC, Chapter 9 (Nutrition and blood), section 9.2.1.2, Oral rehydration therapy. Antimotility drugs not recommended in children under 12 years of age

25 A
See MEP 38, section 3.7.7. Temazepam prescriptions are only valid for 28 days (4 weeks)

26 D
See MEP 38, section 3.7.7. Once daily is a frequency but does not state a dose, i.e. how many tablets to take

27 A
See MEP 38, section 3.7.2. Repeats are not allowed for schedules 2 and 3; instalment prescriptions are required

28 B
See BNF, Chapter 5 (Infections), section 5.1. Table 1 states that clarithromycin can be used in those with penicillin allergy. Note the presence of beta-lactam rings in cephalosporin and carbapenem structures

29 D
See NICE Clinical Guidance 127. ACE inhibitors are a first-line therapy in Caucasian patients under the age of 55. Low-cost angiotensin receptor blockers may be used as a first-line therapy but candesartan is not available as a generic drug, unlike losartan or valsartan

30 D
See BNF, Chapter 2 (Cardiovascular system), section 2.5.5.1. ACE inhibitors may cause profound first-dose hypotension so the patient should take the first dose at bedtime to avoid falls

31 B
See BNF, Chapter 2 (Cardiovascular system), section 2.5.5.1. ACE inhibitors can cause persistent dry cough, which can affect sleep

32 D
See BNF, Chapter 2 (Cardiovascular system), section 2.12. Atorvastatin is a longer-acting statin so may be taken at any time of day. Compare the dosing instructions in monographs for simvastatin and atorvastatin

33 E
Patients suffering diarrhoea after returning from travel abroad should be advised to see their GP for further investigations

34 A
See RPS support documents on Medicines Optimisation

35 A
See BNF, Chapter 2 (Cardiovascular system), section 2.2.3. Amiloride is the only potassium-sparing diuretic listed

36 B
See BNF, Chapter 2 (Cardiovascular system), section 2.2.2. Furosemide can be given twice a day but its duration of action is 6 hours. Therefore, it should not usually be given any later than 4 pm

37 C
See BNF, Chapter 2 (Cardiovascular system), section 2.2.1. Thiazide diuretics may precipitate gout

38 D
See MEP 38, section 3.7.11. Keeping a running balance is best practice, and not a legal requirement

39 B
Martindale: The Complete Drug Reference contains international brand names

40 A
See MEP 38, section 3.6. The address of the prescriber is not needed, only their name

41 C
Fridge temperatures can range between 2°C and 8°C

42 C
See BNF, Chapter 4 (Central nervous system), section 4.2.3, Drugs used for mania and hypomania, Lithium, serum concentrations. See list of overdose signs and symptoms

43 D
See NICE Clinical Guidance 66 and 87. Metformin is first-line therapy for both normal weight and overweight patients

44 B
See BNF, Chapter 6 (Endocrine system), section 6.1.2.2. Hypokalaemia is not a listed side-effect of metformin

45 E
See Drug Tariff part XVIIIB. Generic sildenafil was removed from the Selective List Scheme requirements in August 2014. However, branded sildenafil (*Viagra*) remained on the list

46 C
See BNF, Chapter 4 (Central nervous system), section 4.3.1. Tricyclic antidepressants can cause anticholinergic side-effects; they can also cause hyponatraemia

47 B
See BNF, Chapter 4 (Central nervous system), section 4.7.2. Side-effects are generally in-line with pharmacological activity. Dose reduction may be needed in hypothyroidism

48 B
See BNF, Chapter 2 (Cardiovascular system), section 2.4. Beta-blockers can interfere with the metabolic and autonomic response to hypoglycaemia

49 A
See BNF, Chapter 2 (Cardiovascular system), section 2.4. Beta-blockers can cause bronchospasm and should be avoided in asthma and COPD patients. The more cardioselective beta-blockers may be used if necessary

50 A
See BNF, Appendix 1. Amiodarone inhibits the metabolism of coumarin anticoagulants

51 C
See BNF, Appendix 1. St John's wort is an enzyme-inducer resulting in increased digoxin metabolism

52 B
See Drug Tariff part XVI. Point 10 contains details of what needs to be included on the prescription in order for *Dianette* to be exempt from charges. Otherwise this is assumed to be used for acne (see BNF, Chapter 13 (Skin), section 13.6.2)

53 E
See BNF, Chapter 13 (Skin), section 13.10.3. Aciclovir cream should be applied to the skin every 4 hours

ANSWERS

MULTIPLE COMPLETION ANSWERS

1 A
See treatment of acute severe asthma (in BTS/SIGN guidelines) or BNFC, Chapter 3 (Respiratory system), section 3.1

2 A
Hypokalaemia can be caused by beta agonist therapy. However, in acute severe asthma, this effect will be potentiated by aminophylline, corticosteroids, diuretics, and hypoxia (see BNF, Chapter 3 (Respiratory system), section 3.1.1)

3 E
Salbutamol syrup is not suitable, and it is advisable that you, as a pharmacist, counsel the patient on the inhaler technique

4 A
All of those listed are side-effects related to salbutamol therapy

5 C
Handwriting requirements for controlled drug prescriptions were removed in 2005. Safe custody applies to schedules 1, 2, and 3 controlled drugs (with some exceptions), and a register entry is required for all schedule 1 and 2 controlled drugs

6 B
The prescription is valid for 28 days from the appropriate date

7 C
The following details are legally required on a FP10-CDF: (i) name, form, strength, and quantity; (ii) handwritten signature; (iii) name, occupation/professional qualification, and address of the premises they are working at; and (iv) the purpose for which the drug is required

8 A
Antimuscarinic drugs can cause side-effects such as blurred vision, dry mouth, constipation, difficulty in micturition, among others

9 C
Cimetidine can reduce the antiplatelet effect of clopidogrel and can also increase the plasma concentration of digoxin

10 C
Ibuprofen is not recommended to be used in those patients on lithium or methotrexate. Not all asthmatics will be sensitive to ibuprofen, hence why it can be given to such patients where appropriate

11 A
All of the items are GSL medications that can be purchased over-the-counter

12 B
An age or date of birth is not legally required unless the age of the person is under 12 years of age

13 E
The warning 'keep out of the reach of children' is needed on the label. Cautionary and warning labels are only needed where one applies to the product

14 E
See MEP 38 guidance on returned medication

15 B
See MEP 38, section 3.5.10. In order to make an emergency connection you must (i) explain the reason for the emergency connection request and advise the operator that it is a life-and-death situation, and (ii) give your name and the name of the premises from which you are calling

16 A
See MEP 38, section 3.3.10.2

17 B
A prescription is not required for an emergency supply at the request of a patient

18 A
See MEP 38 guidance and GPhC standards of conduct and ethics

ANSWERS

19 C
Labelling requirements for an emergency supply are the same as for a normal supply, except that the dispensing label must specify the words 'emergency supply'

20 A
Cautionary and warning labels 8 and 10 are required with long-term and high-dose corticosteroids. It is also advisable to tell patients to carry their blue steroid card and to rinse their mouth after using the product

21 B
Flushing and ankle oedema are two known side-effects of calcium-channel blocking agents

22 D
Chlorphenamine is a sedating antihistamine

23 B
Alcohol-containing products should be avoided while on metronidazole

24 A
All reactions as listed should be reported

25 A
A black triangle drug is relatively new to the market, intensively monitored, and all ADRs should be reported via the yellow card reporting scheme

26 A
All statements regarding codeine are true. See MHRA and EMA 2012 guidance

27 A
See MEP 38 guidance and/or a law and ethics textbook. Morphine sulfate 10 mg/5 mL oral solution is a CD Inv POM and so an emergency supply can be made provided the conditions for such a supply are met

28 B
Aminophylline and amiodarone are known to affect thyroid function

29 C
Mrs JM should continue her allopurinol as she was already on it when the acute attack started. See BNF, Chapter 10, section 10.1.4 for information related to colcichine dosing and side-effects.

30 B
NSAIDs are linked to stomach ulcers. There is also a weak link suggesting corticosteroids (such as prednisolone) are also linked with peptic ulcers and perforation

31 B
Aspirin and NSAIDs are known to interact with methotrexate

32 B
Carbamazepine and NSAIDS are known to interact with lithium

33 D
See GPhC guidance on consent and confidentiality

34 A
Hydrocortisone bought over-the-counter should not be used for longer than 7 days without seeking medical attention. The cream should be applied liberally (sometimes termed as sparingly or thinly), and one fingertip unit of cream is equivalent to an application covering both hands

35 C
Options 2 and 3 are significant interactions that either require a change of drug or close careful monitoring

36 C
See GPhC 'standards for pharmacy owners and superintendent pharmacists of retail pharmacy businesses' (September 2010), PAGB 'medicines advertising codes', and PAGB 'guidelines on consumer protection and public relations'.

37 D
Magnesium-containing preparations can cause diarrhoea

38 B
ACEIs are started at night-time to avoid the risk of postural hypotension

39 E
Either an NMS or a MUR can be undertaken at any one time – it is not permissible to do both. The request for an NMS can be at the request of a patient, prescriber, or hospital pharmacist, and is therefore not confined to hospital pharmacy

40 D
Proton pump inhibitors are known to cause atypical femoral or hip fractures

41 E
Antimuscarininc agents can be used to dry-up secretions (e.g. respiratory secretions, hypersalivation, and hyperhidrosis)

42 A
All said points apply to counselling a patient on warfarin

43 C
Loop diuretics and antidepressants can cause hyponatraemia

44 B
Digoxin toxicity can manifest as nausea, vomiting, bradycardia, among others

45 B
Bisoprolol and carvedilol are licensed for use in heart failure

46 C
See MEP 38 guidance on the supply of POMs

47 A
Computer-generated prescriptions must be in English and can have a printed or handwritten date. Any alterations must be countersigned by the prescriber

48 E
The strength and form is legally required on the prescription for any drug

49 B
Refer to RPS guidance on the supply of EHC

50 D
Beta-blockers are contraindicated in asthma

CLASSIFICATION ANSWERS

1 A
Xerophthalmia is characterised by excessive dryness of the conjunctiva and cornea. It may be caused by a deficiency in vitamin A

2 E

3 B

4 C

5 A

6 C
Calcium levels drop in severe diabetic ketoacidosis

7 D

8 E
Zinc is a cofactor in many enzymatic reactions essential to the synthesis of RNA and DNA

9 D

10 A
Isosorbide mononitrate (nitrates cause vasodilation, which can trigger headache)

11 E

12 C

13 B
Champix tablets may cause drowsiness. Do not operate heavy machinery

14 A

15 C

16 D

17 E

18 A

19 B

20 D

21 B
Penicillin V: to be taken an hour before food or on an empty stomach

22 D
Ciprofloxacin: do not take indigestion remedies or medications containing zinc or iron

23 C

24 B

25 C

26 C

27 B

28 B
Tiaprofenic acid is an NSAID. Common class side-effects of NSAIDs include diarrhoea and gastrointestinal irritation

29 B
Haloperidol is a typical antipsychotic. Typical antipsychotics are associated with tardive dyskinesia

30 C

31 A

32 E

33 B
Hyponatraemia predisposes to lithium toxicity

34 A

35 A
Reye's syndrome is a rare but serious condition that causes swelling in the liver and brain. The exact cause is unknown but has been associated with the use of aspirin in children suffering from viral illness. Reye's syndrome most often affects children and teenagers recovering from a viral infection and who may also have a metabolic disorder, and may occur without use of aspirin. However, children and teenagers recovering from chickenpox or flu-like symptoms should never take aspirin

36 E

37 B

38 C

39 C

40 A

41 A

42 A

43 C

44 E

45 D

46 D

47 B

48 A

49 E

50 B
Liquid paraffin is not widely used as it is associated with lipoid pneumonia

51 A

52 B

53 E
Lactulose is an osmotic laxative that can also be used to treat hepatic encephalopathy

54 B

55 B

56 D
Diamorphine must be recorded in a controlled drugs register

57 B

58 B

59 E
Dexamethasone is a potent corticosteroid, and as such is associated with immunosuppression

60 B

61 A

62 A

63 A

64 B

65 B

STATEMENT ANSWERS

1 A
See BNF, Chapter 2 (Cardiovascular system), section 2.4

2 B
See BNF, Appendix 1, Interactions

3 E
See BNF, Chapter 6 (Endocrine system), section 6.1.2

4 C
See BNF, Chapter 7 (Obstetrics, gynaecology, and urinary-tract disorders), section 7.3.1

5 A
See BNF, Chapter 4 (Central nervous system), section 4.3

6 C
See BNF, Chapter 10 (Musculoskeletal and joint diseases), section 10.1.1

7 E
See BNF, Chapter 2 (Cardiovascular system), section 2.12

8 A
See BNF, Chapter 5 (Infections), section 5.1.9

9 A
See BNF, Chapter 5 (Infections), section 5.1.4

10 B
See BNF, Appendix 4, Intravenous additives

11 B
See BNF, Chapter 3 (Respiratory system), section 3.1.3

12 B
See BNF, Chapter 2 (Cardiovascular system), section 2.4

ANSWERS

13 C
See BNF, Chapter 2 (Cardiovascular system), section 2.2.2

14 B
See BNF, Chapter 6 (Endocrine system), section 6.6

15 A
See BNF, Appendix 1, Interactions

16 D
See BNF, Chapter 2 (Cardiovascular system), section 2.3.2

17 B
See BNF, Chapter 4 (Central nervous system), section 4.8.1

18 B
See BNF, Chapter 4 (Central nervous system), section 4.7.2

19 A

20 A

21 A

22 C

23 A

24 B

25 C

26 E

27 E

28 C

29 D

30 E

31 A

32 E

33 C

34 D

35 B

36 E

37 B

38 A

39 E

40 B

41 C
Co-amoxiclav 250/125 mg tablets are allowed on the Dental Practitioners' Formulary; the 500/125 mg strength is not allowed. The non-proprietary name of a drug or preparation should ideally be used for NHS prescriptions but brand names are also legally valid

42 B

43 E

44 A

45 D

46 C
See BNF, Chapter 5 (Infections), section 5.4.1. There may be a risk of harm to the fetus with some antimalarial medicines

47 B
See BNF, Chapter 3 (Respiratory system), section 3.6

48 D

49 E
See BNF, Prescribing for children

50 A

Calculation answers

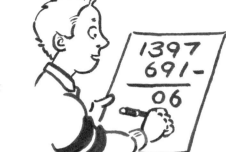

1 E

The BNF monograph for dantrolene specifies that the cumulative maximum is 10 mg/kg

2 B

See BNF, Chapter 7 (Obstetrics, gynaecology, and urinary-tract disorders), section 7.2.1. The drug monograph specifies this is a 0.01% cream, which is 0.01 g in 100 g; hence, 0.008 g (= 8 mg) in a single 80-g tube

3 E

$(6 \times 5) + (4 \times 3) + (2 \times 3) + [(17 \times 1)/2] = 30 + 12 + 6 + 8.5 = 56.5$. As we cannot give half a tablet, the nearest practical amount is 57 tablets

4 E

$t_{1/2} = 4$ hours; $C_{ss} = 19.6$ hours. Therefore, $19.6/4 = 4.9$, and hence, approximately 5 half-lives

5 C

$100 \times 0.84 = 84$ mL of TPN per day; hence, $84/24 = 3.5$ mL/hour

6 A

1 in 100 solution when diluted tenfold will provide a 1 in 1000 solution. This tells us we need to add 1 part of solution A to 9 parts of diluent

ANSWERS

167

7 C
100 mL of omeprazole 10 mg/5 mL contains 200 mg of omeprazole

Millimoles = mass(mg)/molecular weight
Millimoles = 200/345 = 0.579 = 0.6 mmol

8 D
Aminophylline injection is an 80 : 20 mixture and so has a bioavail-ability of 0.8 (i.e. 80%)

400 × 0.8 = 320 mg

9 D
Using the alligation method it can be found that there are 40 parts in total. Of these parts, 38 parts are for the 10% glucose, and 2 parts are for the 50% glucose. Hence, we will need 38/40 × 500 = 475 mL of glucose 10%, and 25 mL of glucose 50%

10 E
See conversion tables in the BNF.

BSA = $\sqrt{\{[110 \times 18]/3600]\}}$
     = $\sqrt{\{1980/3600\}}$
     = $\sqrt{\{1980/3600\}}$
BSA = $\sqrt{0.55}$

i.e. 0.74 × 0.74 = ≈0.55
Or see table in BNFC Appendix for Body surface area in children

11 D
The exact number is 24 but the product should be supplied as a special container of 30 capsules.
2 × 250 nanogram capsules, thrice weekly for four weeks = 24

12 D
6 tablets daily for 2 months i.e. 6 × 60 days = 360 tablets. See BNF, Chapter 5 (Infections), section 5.1.9

13 A

7.5 mg/kg for a 20-kg child is 150 mg/day, which would be 50 mg/dose. Therefore, 80 mg in 2 mL = 8 mg in 0.2 mL = 1 mg in 0.025 mL; hence, 0.025 mL ×50 = 1.25 mL

14 A

0.05% = 0.05 g in 100 g

      = 0.005 g in 10 g

      = 0.015 g in 30 g = 15 mg

15 D

150 mg in 5 mL = 225 mg in 7.5 mL
7.5 × 4 = 30 mL (daily dose)
30 mL ×14 = 420 mL

16 B

20% w/v = 20 g in 100 mL
2 g in 10 mL
6 g in 30 mL (*x*)
0.6 g in 3 mL (*y*)
(*x*) + (*y*) = 6.6 g in 33 mL

17 C

1 drop into both eyes, five times daily = 10 drops per day
28 days = 280 drops
280 drops/15 = 18.67 mL
You would supply two full 10 mL bottles for Mrs D

18 D

Enteric-coated tablets are not available as 1-mg strength, so answers A and C are not possible. The tablets are not easily split (and the enteric coating would be pointless) so only using 5 mg tablets would not be appropriate.

19 E

To make Double-Strength Peppermint Water BP from Concentrated Peppermint Water BP, it is necessary to dilute 1 part concentrate with 19 parts water.

20 B
The maximum dose is 1.5 mg over 24 hours i.e. 6 × 250 mcg tablets; 10 × 250 mcg tablets would be 2.5 mg, which would be an overdose

21 C
Atripla contains efavirenz 600 mg + emtricitabine 200 mg + tenofovir disproxil 245 mg as a fixed dose combination. With the options given, the only way of achieving this combination at this dose is to choose 30 × *Truvada* tablets (emtricitabine 200 mg + tenofovir disproxil 245 mg) and 90 × *Sustiva* 200 mg capsules (taking three capsules daily would provide efavirenz 600 mg)

22 A
The recommended quantity for both arms is 30 g to 60 g for 2 weeks; for 1 month this would be about 60 g to 120 g for both arms. Mr E just needs sufficient for the left arm so an amount between 30 g and 60 g would be appropriate

23 C
See conversion tables in the BNF.
1 foot (ft) = 304.8 mm and 1 inch (in) = 25.4 mm, therefore 4 ft 11 in = 1.498 m
13 st = 82.55 kg and 1 lb = 0.45 kg, therefore 13 st 1 lb = 83 kg
Thus, BMI (kg/m^2) = (83/1.498)/1.498 = 36.988 kg/m^2
Or, with rounding = (83/1.50)/1.50 = 36.889 kg/m^2
Note: Calculating as 83/(1.50 × 1.50) will also give you 36.899 kg/m^2

24 A
Calculate target weight: (24 × 1.5) × 1.5 = 54 kg
Calculate weight to be lost: 83-54 = 29 kg
Use conversation tables in the BNF.
25.4 kg = 4 st, and 3.63 kg = 8 lbs, therefore 4 st 8 lbs = 29.03 kg

25 C
The Cockcroft and Gault formula is found in the prescribing in renal impairment guidance in the BNF.
Note: The constant will be 1.23 as this is a male patient.
CrCl = [(140-60) × 80 × 1.23]/200 = 39.36 mL/minute
It is possible to calculate this without rounding the constant to 1.25

26 B

First convert the height into cm: 180 cm.

Calculate values inside square brackets: $[180 \times 80] = 14\,400$.

Then, within the round brackets: $(14\,400/3600) = 4$.

Power of a half $(X^{0.5})$ is the same as performing a square root.

Therefore, BSA: $\sqrt{4} = 2\,m^2$

27 B

For every $1\,m^2$ of BSA the patient should receive 1.8 mg busulfan

Therefore: $1.8 \times 2 = 3.6\,mg$

28 E

The patient is receiving 120 mg morphine each day. Therefore, the rescue dose is $120/6 = 20\,mg$

29 C

See BNF, Chapter 4 (Central nervous system), section 4.7.2. *Oramorph* oral solution is 10 mg/5 mL, and therefore 20 mg/10 mL

30 D

The total *Zomorph* dose is 140 mg, so the rescue dose is (140/7) 20 mg. Therefore, the patient receives 160 mg to 180 mg morphine daily.

Use the morphine-to-fentanyl conversion table in the prescribing in palliative care section of the BNF

31 D

Phenytoin capsules contain the sodium salt, while the suspension is the base.

Therefore, 100 mg of capsules is equal to 90 mg suspension, and thus, the daily dose is 180 mg.

See BNF, Chapter 4 (Central nervous system), section 4.8.1. The strength of suspension is 30 mg/5 mL

Therefore, 30 mL of suspension is needed ($30\,mg/5\,mL \times 6 = 180\,mg /30\,mL$)

32 D

The equation of the line needs to be rearranged:

$x = (y - 0.05)/0.01$

Therefore: $x = (0.55 - 0.05)/0.01 = 50\,mg/mL$

33   **D**
See BNF, Chapter 5 (Infections), section 5.4.1. *Malarone* should be
started 1–2 days before entering an endemic area and continued for
a week after leaving. The patient is not at risk while they are in
Hanoi. Therefore, Miss L should receive 23 tablets (2 + 14 + 7)

34   **D**
See BNF, Chapter 2 (Cardiovascular system), section 2.8.1. See also
conversion tables in the BNF.
Initial heparin loading dose for pulmonary embolism is 75 mg/kg.
The patient's ideal body weight is 50 + (2.3 × 10) = 73 kg
Therefore, the dose is 75 × 73 = 5475 units

35   **A**
See BNF, Chapter 2 (Cardiovascular system), section 2.8.1. Continu-
ous infusion for pulmonary embolism calculated at 18 units/kg/hour.
Therefore, 18 × 73 = 1314 units/hour

36   **E**
200 microlitres of culture was grown so need to convert to 1 mL i.e.
multiply each CFU count by 5.
Convert the grown samples to original culture, i.e. multiply each
value by the respective dilution factor.
Add all the values together, then divide by six (the number of
samples):
e.g. with plate 1: 12 × 5 = 60, then 60 × 10 000 = 600 000. This is
the original culture CFU count, and therefore:
Average CFUs = (600 000 + 500 000 + 550 000 + 550 000 +
600 000 + 625 000)/6 = 570 830 CFUs

37   **B**
See BNF, Appendix 4.Use the list of intravenous additives to find the
concentration.
Not fluid-restricted so should reconstitute to no stronger than
5 mg/mL.
Thus, 1000 mg (single dose)/5 mg/mL = 200 mL

38 C
See BNF, Appendix 4. For doses over 500 mg the rate should be no faster than 10 mg/minute.
Work out the number of minutes: 1000 mg (single dose)/10 = 100 minutes
Work out the rate: 200 mL /100 minutes = 2 mL/minute

39 D
See BNF, Chapter 2 (Cardiovascular system), section 2.8.2. Warfarin tablets are available in 500 mcg, 1 mg, 3 mg, and 5 mg strengths only. Twenty-eight 3-mg tablets and 14 1-mg tablets will allow Mr B to achieve the desired 3-mg and 4-mg doses in the fewest number of tablets, and without breaking tablets.
Note: these tablets are not stated as being scored, so splitting should be avoided where possible

40 B
See conversion tables in the BNF.
Place the numbers you have been supplied into the equation given:

Total iron dose $= 56 \times ([14-9] \times 2.4) + 500 = 1196$ mg

Note: If you add the constant (500) before multiplying by the body weight you will get this wrong.

41 C
Maximum dose = 200 mg, so the number of doses is 1196 / 200 = 5.98 doses.
Therefore, it will take 2 weeks to infuse six (5.98) doses as no more than three infusions per week can be administered

42 B
Ideal body weight $= 50 + (2.5 \times 5) = 61.5$ kg
DigCl $= (0.06 \times 49) + (0.05 \times 61.5) = 2.94 + 3.075 = 6.015$, rounded to 6.02 L/hour

43 D
Rearranging the equation will give:

Dose $= (C_{pss} \times DigCl \times t) / F$

F is 1 for IV administration, therefore:

Dose $= C_{pss} \times DigCl \times t$

If $C_{pss} = 1.5$: Dose $= 1.5 \times 6 \times 24 = 216$ mcg
If $C_{pss} = 2.0$: Dose $= 2.0 \times 6 \times 24 = 288$ mcg
If aiming directly for the middle of the range (1.75): Dose $= 1.75 \times 6 \times 24 = 252$ mcg

44 C
Number of vials $= (3 \times 60)/100 = 180/100 = 1.8$ vials.
As whole vials are needed, round-up to 2.0

45 E
See BNFC, Chapter 6 (Endocrine system), section 6.3.2. Use the glucocorticoid conversion table.
800 mcg methylprednisolone $= 1$ mg prednisolone
Thus, 8 mg methylprednisolone $= 10$ mg prednisolone
1 mg methylprednisolone $= 1.25$ mg prednisolone
Therefore, total dose $= 40 \times 1.25 = 50$ mg prednisolone

46 C
The average weight of a 7-year-old is given as 23 kg (see BNFC).
Using the dosing regimen given:

Dose $= 0.5$ mg/kg $\times 23$ kg $= 11.5$ mg

See BNF, Chapter 2 (Cardiovascular system), section 2.2.2. The furosemide monograph states a dilution to 1–2 mg/mL should be used. Therefore, $11.5/2 = 5.75$ mL

47 D
Molecular weight of potassium chloride (KCl) = 39 + 35.5 = 74.5
Moles = mass/molecular weight; rearrange to give: mass = moles ×
molecular weight
Thus, mass needed per infusion bag = 40 mmols ×74.5 = 2980 mg
For 15% w/v vials = 15 000 mg per 100 mL = 150 mg/mL = 1 mg
in 0.00666 mL
Therefore, 0.00666 × 2980 = 19.8666 mL of KCl solution

48 D
The patient needs 240 mcg/minute (3 × 80). Infusion bags contain
160 000 mcg in 100 mL (1600 mcg per 1 mL).
Thus, 240 mcg in 0.150 mL, and therefore, 0.15 × 60 = 9 mL/hour

49 E
The final solution is 0.05% w/v = 0.05 g in 100 mL = 0.1 g (i.e.
100 mg) in 200 mL. The 100 mg came from 5 mL of the original
solution. Therefore, 100/5 = 20 mg/mL

50 A
See BNF, Chapter 13 (Skin), section 13.10.2. See the formula given
under Benzoic acid (Whitfield's ointment).
5% (excess) of 60 g is 3 g, so need to make 63 g in total.
Benzoic acid is 6%, therefore: 63/100 × 6 = 3.78 g
Salicylic acid is 3%, therefore: 63/100 × 3 = 1.89 g

51 B
Note: You need to use the allegation method here, as it is not as
simple as adding the assumed amount of solid.
Need to make 15 g: 15 g/1.5 parts = 10 g per part.
Therefore, 0.5 × 10 = 5 g of 1% cream, 1 × 10 = 10 g of 2.5%
cream

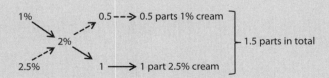

52 C

The allegation method can be used here again.

Thus, the 2% cream makes 95 parts of final 98 parts: 50 / 95 = 0.526 g/part.

Therefore, 3 parts ×0.526 g/part = 1.579 g salicylic acid to add.

The answer can be checked as follows: ([1.00 + 1.58] / [50 + 1.58]) × 100 = 5.00%

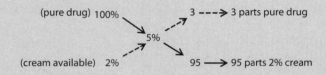

MULTIPLE COMPLETION ANSWERS

1 B
See BNF, Chapter 1 (Gastro-intestinal system), section 1.1.2. Options 1 and 2 contain 3.1 and 3 mmol sodium per 5 mL, respectively. Option 3 contains 2.13 mmol sodium per 5 mL

2 C
See BNF, Chapter 9 (Nutrition and blood), section 9.6.4. Option 1 contains 200 units of vitamin D, whereas options 2 and 3 contain 400 units per unit dose.

3 A
See BNFC, Appendix 4, for details

4 B
See BNFC, Chapter 5 (Infections), section 5.1.2.2. The drug monograph specifies a dose of 10–20 mg/kg, which is normally every 8 hours. However, in renal impairment with an eGFR of the range 26–50mL/minute/1.73m^2, the frequency is reduced to every 12 hours.

5 C
See individual drug monographs in BNFC. For option 2, the dose is 800 mg five times daily for 7 days, and for option 3, the dose is 600 mg once daily

ANSWERS

6 E

3 only is correct:

1 Each ampoule should be diluted to 500 mL. A 5 mL ampoule contains 800 mg dopamine. If diluted to 400 mL, this gives 800 mg in 400 mL; 2 mg/mL in the resulting infusion

2 In 1 minute the patient should receive 240 mcg of dopamine, based on a body weight of 80 kg, therefore:

3 240 mcg × 60 minutes = 14 400 mcg, equivalent to 14.4 mg/hour

4 The dose should be 240 mcg per minute. As 240 mcg = 0.24 mg:

1 mL of solution contains 1.6 mg
0.1 mL of solution contains 0.16 mg
0.05 mL of solution contains 0.08 mg.

Therefore, 0.15mL of solution contains 0.24mg – the volume for the dose per minute

7 C

2 and 3 only are correct:

1 A child of this weight is likely to be under 12 years old if the weight is normal so doxycycline would be contraindicated.

2 For a 25-kg child, the weekly dose of mefloquine is 187.5 mg. This can be started 3 weeks prior to travel, taken for 1 week away and then continued for 4 weeks after leaving the risk area, giving a total of 8 weeks of therapy. As 187.5 mg is three-quarters of a 250 mg tablet, then 8 × 0.75 = 6 tablets

3 For a 25-kg child, the dose of *Malarone* paediatric tablets is two tablets daily. This can be started 1 day before travel, taken each day during the trip, and then continued for 7 days after return, which amounts to 15 days in total. Two tablets daily for 15 days = 30 tablets

CLASSIFICATION ANSWERS

1 E

2 A

3 D

4 C
See BNF, Chapter 5 (Infections), section 5.1.1.3. Normal dose volume given at 12-hourly intervals

5 E
See BNF, Chapter 5 (Infections), section 5.2.1. Dose is 3–5 mg/kg; maximum dose is 5 mg/kg.
$18 \times 5 = 90\,\text{mg} = 9\,\text{mL}$ of suspension

6 C
1.5 g in 100 mL;
0.15 g in 10 mL;
0.9 g in 60 mL

7 E
10% solution of 90 mL (45 mL starting solution plus an equal volume) = 9 g

8 D
There are 1600 units per capsule.
5 capsules per day = 8000 units
8000×28 days $= 224\,000$ units

9 E
Lantus injections contain 100 units/mL $= 100\,000$ units/L $= 240\,000$ units in 2.4 L

10 C
400 units per tablet ×60 = 24 000 units

11 C
Emulsifying wax is 30% w/w of Emulsifying Ointment BP.
0.3 × 15 kg = 4.5 kg

12 B
White soft paraffin is 50% w/w of Emulsifying Ointment BP.
0.5 × 6 kg = 3 kg

13 B
Dose:

360 mg per 24 hours
15 mg per hour
0.25 mg per minute
Concentration:
360 mg/20 mL
18 mg/mL
4 hours and 27 minutes = 267 minutes
267 minutes ×0.25 mg = 66.75 mg
66.75 mg/18 = 3.7 mL approximately

14 E
7 hours and 58 minutes = 478 minutes
478 minutes ×0.25 mg = 119.5 mg
119.5 mg/18 = 6.6 mL approximately

15 D
See BNFC, Chapter 4 (Central nervous system), section 4.7.1. Post-operative pain in children over 8 years of age is dosed at 15–20 mg/kg every 4–6 hours.
Therefore, 26 × 20 = 520 mg every 4–6 hours

16 **C**
See BNFC, Chapter 4 (Central nervous system), section 4.7.1. IV
dose for children weighing 10–50 kg is 15 mg/kg every 4–6 hours.
Thus, $34 \times 15 = 510$ mg
However, regular haemodialysis indicates renal insufficiency so dura-
tion should be extended as per BNFC.

17 **A**
See BNFC, Chapter 4 (Central nervous system), section 4.7.1. The
correct gestational age is 28 weeks, therefore the dose is calculated
as 10–15 mg/kg every 8–12 hours. Use conversion tables in BNFC
to find out the weight (around 3.5 kg).
Thus, $3.5 \times 10 = 35$ mg, while $3.5 \times 15 = 52.5$ mg.
Therefore, 50 mg every 12 hours is most appropriate

18 **D**
See BNFC, Chapter 4 (Central nervous system), section 4.7.1. Similar
to question 15. Find the weight in BNFC as 32 kg.
Thus, $32 \times 15 = 480$ mg, while $32 \times 20 = 640$ mg.
Therefore, 500 mg every 4–6 hours is most appropriate

ANSWERS

STATEMENT ANSWERS

1 A
Statement 1: 20 mg/12 hours = 1.66 mg/hour or approximately 1.7 mg/hour.
Statement 2: BNF, Chapter 4 (Central nervous system), section 4.9.1 specifies that the usual maintenance rate via this route is 1–4 mg/hour (15–60 mcg/kg/hour)

2 D
Statement 1 is false since one bottle of *Nutrini® Multi Fibre Liquid* is 200 mL in volume and contains 200 kcal of energy. Statement 2 is true if you divide the energy values provided in the ACBS listings in the BNFC.

3 A
Both statements are true and statement 2 explains why the drug is dosed as in statement 1.
600 mg over 90 minutes + (12.5 × 2 × 10.5 over the remaining 10½ hours) = 600 + 262.5 mg = 862.5 mg or 863 mg

4 A
Both statements are true and statement 2 explains why the rate is at 52 mL hour (i.e. 52 × 24 = ~1250 mL).
See BNFC, Chapter 9 (Nutrition and blood), section 9.2.2.1, table entitled 'Fluid requirements for children over 1 month'
100 mL/kg for 1st 10 kg 1000 mL
+50 mL/kg for next 10 kg 250 mL

5 A
A 1-to-1 dilution is required to produce a solution that is half the strength of the original.
For example, adding 10 mL of the 8.4% solution to 10 mL water for injection will give 20 mL of a 4.2% solution

6 A
A 3-week-old baby born at 28 weeks' of gestation has a gestational age of 31 weeks. For a child of this age, the correct dose of vancomycin in this instance would be 15 mg/kg every 24 hours, i.e. 30 mg vancomycin.
The dose must be given over at least 60 minutes so the fastest possible rate would be:

30 mg/60 minutes
5 mg/10 minutes
0.5 mg/minute

7 D
See BNF, Chapter 3 (Respiratory system), section 3.1, Management of acute asthma. For moderate acute asthma the recommended upper dose for salbutamol over 1 hour would be:
Nebuliser
5 mg salbutamol repeated at intervals at least 20 minutes apart. During 1 hour the dosage would be 5 mg ×3 = 15 mg
Metered-dose inhaler 10 puffs × 100 mcg = 1 mg inhaled every 10 minutes. During 1 hour the maximum under this dosage would be 6 mg

ANSWERS

Index

abbreviations used in prescribing, Latin, 21
Abidec, children, 39
accuracy checking, prescription, 49
ACEI. *See* angiotensin-converting enzyme inhibitor
aciclovir (*Zovirax*) topical cream
  cold sore, 58
  dosage, 58
aciclovir tablets, dose calculation, 109
acne, drugs treating, 75
acromegaly, drug(s) for treating, 28
acute asthma, 59–60
  salbutamol inhaler, dose calculation, 101, 116
acute myocardial infarction
  cardiac enzymes and biomarkers, 25
  contraindicated drugs, 28
  diagnosing, 25
acute porphyria
  antibiotics prescribing, 1–2
  children, 1–2
  contraception, 17
  emergency contraception, 17
  Levonelle, 17
  staphylococcal skin infection, 1–2
Adcal-D3 tablets, calculation, 112
adherence to drug treatment, children, 17
adrenaline (epinephrine), 28, 29
adrenaline (epinephrine), intramuscular
  anaphylactic reactions, 15
  children, 15
  dosage, 15
  nut allergy, 15
adverse reactions
  co-cyprindiol (Dianette), 65
  Dianette (co-cyprindiol), 65

reporting, 65, 87
statements, 87
Tegaderm hydrocolloid dressings, 87
alcoholic patients, drugs of concern, 47
alfacalcidol, calculation, 92
allergy. *See also* anaphylactic reactions
  children, 39
  nut allergy, 15
  penicillin allergy, 75
  sorbic acid, 9
  statements, 86
allopurinol
  drug interactions, 26
  gout, 66
Ambisome
  diluents, 12
  infusion method, 12
amiloride
  side-effects, 73
  statements, 81
aminoglycosides, statements, 79
aminophylline injection, calculation, 91
amiodarone
  advice, 11
  counselling, 11
  monitoring, 9
  side-effects, 29
  statements, 81
  Wolff-Parkinson-White syndrome, 11
amiodarone hydrochloride, statements, 73
amitriptyline, 28
  depression, 56
  side-effects, 56
  statements, 82
amlodipine
  repeat prescriptions, 2–3
  side-effects, 64

amoxicillin suspension, dose
    calculation, 109
anaemia associated with chronic renal
    failure, 27
anaerobic infections, drugs treating, 75
analgesics
    back pain, 6
    concurrent use with methotrexate,
        3–4
    pregnancy, 6–7
anaphylactic reactions. *See also* allergy
    adrenaline (epinephrine),
        intramuscular, 15
    children, 5, 15
    drug(s) for treating, 28
    egg-based products, 5
    nut allergy, 15
    vaccinations, 5
angiotensin-converting enzyme
    inhibitor (ACEI), counselling, 68
antibiotics prescribing
    acute porphyria, 1–2
    children, 2, 8
    glucose-6-phosphate dehydrogenase
        deficiency, 8
    haemolysis risk, 8
    staphylococcal skin infection, 2
    urinary-tract infection, 8
antibiotics, cautionary labels, 73
antidepressants, statements, 79
antidiabetic medications
    overweight patients, 28
    pregnancy, 22
antihyperglycaemic drugs, type 2
    diabetes, 55
antimalarial medicines
    pregnancy, 87
    statements, 109
antipsychotics
    atypical, 32
    side-effects, 20
    weight gain side-effect, 20
anti-rheumatic drugs, washout
    procedures, 20
antitussive drug, 75
antiviral agents, cytomegalovirus
    (CMV), 16
apomorphine continuous subcutaneous
    maintenance infusion pump,
    statements, 114

apraclonidine, indications, 27
aqueous cream, 34
arginine, statements, 115
arterial blood gas results, acute severe
    asthma, 59–60
arthritis. *See also* rheumatoid arthritis
    methotrexate, 3–4
    peptic ulcer, 44
aspirin. *See also* salicylic acid cream
    repeat prescriptions, 2
    statements, 79
asthma
    acute, 59–60, 101, 116
    arterial blood gas results, 59
    children, 37, 39, 59–60
    contraindicated drugs, 70
    flu vaccinations, 37
    propranolol, 57
    salbutamol inhaler, 60, 84
    salbutamol inhaler, dose calculation,
        102, 116
    salbutamol syrup, 60
    smoking cessation, 84
    statements, 59
    Ventolin Evohaler, 37
atenolol
    conditions for caution, 9, 57
    diabetes, 57
    emergency supply, 64
athlete's foot, drugs treating, 77
atorvastatin
    hypertension, 52
    statements, 79
atrial fibrillation, warfarin, 37
Atripla tablets, calculation, 95
atropine eye drops, Parkinson's disease
    symptoms alleviated by, 69
audit, statements, 83
Augmentin tablets, statements, 85–86
azathioprine, drug interactions, 26

babies. *See also* neonates
    eczema, 24
    Trimovate cream, 24
baby milks, prohibited promotion
    activities, 67
back pain
    analgesics, 6
    pregnancy, 6–7

baldness, drugs treating male pattern, 76–77
beclometasone 100 mcg inhaler
 advice, 64
 side-effects, 64
Benadryl 8 mg capsules, 30
bendroflumethiazide
 drug interactions, 26
 side-effects, 73
benzodiazepines, withdrawal, 25
beta-blockers, heart failure, 69
Betnovate cream, eczema, 10
bisoprolol
 drug interactions, 26
 statements, 72
blood disorders, drugs causing, 19
body mass index (BMI), calculation, 95
body surface area (BSA), calculations, 92, 96–97
bone marrow depression, cytotoxic drugs, 23
breastfeeding, contraindicated drugs, 7, 18
Bricanyl respules 5 mg/2mL, side-effects, 30
BSA. *See* body surface area
buprenorphine 2.5 mcg patches, destruction, 13
buprenorphine, indications, 27
Buscopan (hyoscine butylbromide) tablets, side-effects, 61
busulfan, calculation, 97
butylated hydroxyanisole, E number, 26

calcium alginate dressings, 36
calcium, statements, 71
cancer drugs. *See* chemotherapy drugs; cytotoxic drugs; palliative care
cannabis, 29
captopril oral liquid, children, 41
carbamazepine, drug interactions, 26
cardiac enzymes and biomarkers, acute myocardial infarction, 25
cardiovascular risk prediction, 13
cautionary labels, 72
 antibiotics, 73
 Champix tablets, 72
 ciprofloxacin, 73
 clarithromycin 250 mg tablets, 27

clarithromycin tablets, 72
doxycycline 100 mg capsules, 27
doxycycline capsules, 72
erythromycin 250 mg tablets, 27
erythromycin coated tablets, 72
flucloxacillin, 73
metoclopramide modified-release capsules, 72
minocycline, 73
nitrofurantoin 100 mg capsules, 27
oxytetracycline 250 mg tablets, 27
penicillin V (phenoxymethylpenicillin), 73
cellulitis, oral antibacterial therapy, 51
cephalosporins, 35
CFUs. *See* colony forming units
Champix tablets, cautionary labels, 72
charges, NHS prescription. *See* NHS prescription charges
chemotherapy drugs. *See also* cytotoxic drugs
 emetogenic drugs, 16
 intrathecal administration, 15
children. *See also* babies; neonates
 Abidec, 39
 acute porphyria, 2
 adherence to drug treatment, 17
 adrenaline (epinephrine), intramuscular, 15
 allergy, 15, 39
 anaphylactic reactions, 15, 48
 antibiotics prescribing, 2, 16
 arginine, statements, 115
 asthma, 15, 39, 60
 captopril oral liquid, 41
 cough, 10
 cough, dry, 46
 diarrhoea, 50
 epinephrine (adrenaline), intramuscular, 15
 flu vaccinations, 37
 fluid replacement, syringe pump calculation, 115
 glucose-6-phosphate dehydrogenase deficiency, 8
 haemolysis risk, 8
 MMR vaccine, 5–6
 nut allergy, 15
 Nutrini® *Multi Fibre Liquid*, statements, 115

children (*continued*)
  paracetamol 120 mg/5 ml oral
    suspension, 36
  pertussis vaccine, withholding, 24
  postoperative anti-inflammatory, 47
  sildenafil, 40
  staphylococcal skin infection, 2
  thyroid hormones, 24
  urinary-tract infection, 8
  vaccinations, 5, 19, 24
  Ventolin Evohaler, 15
chlorhexidine solution, calculation, 106
chlorphenamine (Piriton) syrup,
    side-effects, 65
chlorpromazine
  clozapine dose equivalence,
    schizophrenia, 9
  drug interactions, 26
cholecalciferol, calculation, 112
cholestatic jaundice, statements, 86
chronic obstructive pulmonary disease
    (COPD)
  oxygen therapy, 87
  statements, 83, 87
ciclosporin, 32
Cilest tablets, FP10 prescriptions, 8
cilostazol, 29
cimetidine tablets, drug interactions, 61
ciprofloxacin, 27
  cautionary labels, 63
citrullinaemia, arginine, statements,
    115
clarithromycin 250 mg tablets,
    cautionary labels, 27
clarithromycin tablets, cautionary
    labels, 72
clinical audits, 38
clobetasol propionate, calculation, 93
clobetasone butyrate 0.05% cream,
    over-the-counter (OTC)
    prescribing, 14
clomipramine, vs phenelzine, 13
Clostridium difficile infection, drugs
    treating, 75
clozapine/chlorpromazine dose
    equivalence, schizophrenia, 9
CMV. *See* cytomegalovirus
co-amoxiclav
  dosage, 111
  statements, 86

co-amoxiclav/co-codamol/co-cyprindiol/
    co-dydramol/co-phenotrope,
  suitability for prescribing, 7
co-cyprindiol (Dianette), adverse
    reactions, 65
codeine phosphate 25 mg/5mL oral
    solution, statements, 26
codeine phosphate, indications, 65–66
colchicine, gout, 66
cold and flu remedies, 75
cold sore, *Zovirax* (aciclovir) topical
    cream, 58
colony forming units (CFUs),
    calculation, 100–101
colour vision disturbance, side-effect,
    29
community pharmacy, good dispensing
    practice, 63
Compound Benzoic Acid Ointment BP,
    calculation, 106
compounding non-sterile products, 106
computer-generated prescriptions,
    statements, 70
concentration of a drug, calculation,
    98–99
conditions for caution
  atenolol, 9, 57
  methotrexate, 4
confidentiality, statements, 83
constipation
  ferrous iron alternatives, 12
  side-effect, 29
  statements, 81
continuing professional development
    (CPD), 39, 44, 50
  statements, 86
contraception. *See also* emergency
    contraception
  acute porphyria, 17
  advice, 25
  effectiveness of methods, 6
  Levonelle, 17, 83
  Microgynon, 25, 45, 63, 79
  oral contraceptive pills, emergency
    supply, 84
  oral contraceptive pills, statements,
    79
controlled drugs
  destruction, 25

exemptions from prescription
requirements, 76
exemptions from safe-custody
requirements, 76
FP10 prescriptions, 60
legislation, 60–61
record requirements, 60–61, 76
schedule 1 controlled drug, 29
schedule 2 controlled drugs, 61
schedules, 51
supplying, 60–61
controlled drugs registers
disposal time, 49
recorded particulars, 54
COPD. *See* chronic obstructive
pulmonary disease
Copegus capsules, dose regimen, 14
corticosteroids. *See also* topical
corticosteroids
prolonged use, 23
side-effects, 23
cough
antitussive drug, 75
children, 24
expectorant drug, 75
pertussis vaccine, 24
cough, dry
children, 46
ramipril alternatives, 10
CPD. *See* continuing professional
development
C-reactive protein, statements, 81
creatinine clearance rate, calculation,
96
cytomegalovirus (CMV), antiviral
agents, 16
cytotoxic drugs, 23, *See also*
chemotherapy drugs, bone marrow
depression

dabigatran etexilate, statements, 72
dantrolene sodium, calculation, 89
demulcent drug, 75
dental prescription, erythromycin
capsules, 40–41
depression
amitriptyline, 56
antidepressants, statements, 79
course of action, 48
rheumatoid arthritis, 48

dermatological preparations
Lyclear Dermal Cream, 4–5
scabies, 4–5
Dermovate cream, calculation, 93
Desmotabs 200 mcg tablets,
side-effects, 30
destruction
buprenorphine 2.5 mcg patches, 13
controlled drugs, 25
dexamfetamine 5 mg tablets, 29
dexrazoxane, licensing, 21
diabetes
antidiabetic medications, 22, 27–28
antihyperglycaemic drugs, 55
atenolol, 57
metformin, 56
overweight patients, 27–28
pregnancy, 22
propranolol, 57
self-monitoring, 22
sildenafil, 7, 56
type 2 diabetes, 22, 55–56
diabetic ketoacidosis, 33
diamorphine subcutaneous infusion, 18
calculation, 113
compatibility with other drugs, 18
dosage, 12
vs morphine sulfate, 12
Dianette (co-cyprindiol), adverse
reactions, 65
diarrhoea
children, 50
course of action, 52
drugs causing, 68, 74
diazepam 10 mg/2mL injection, 29
diazepam 5 mg tablets, dosing
instructions, 51
diclofenac 2.32% gel, over-the-counter
(OTC) prescribing, 14
DigiFab
digoxin toxicity, 104
dose calculation, 103–4
digitalis toxicity
digoxin, 20
electrolyte imbalances, 20
heart failure, 20
dignity, statements, 83
digoxin
calculation, 94
DigiFab dose calculation, 104

digoxin (*continued*)
  digitalis toxicity, 20
  dose calculation, 103–4
  drug interactions, 57
  electrolyte imbalances, 20, 48
  heart failure, 20
  St John's wort, 57
  statements, 81
  toxicity, 47–48, 104
  toxicity signs, 69
dilution calculations, 91, 94, 105, 115
dinoprostone, contraindicated
    circumstances, 23
disclosure, patient information, 67
disulfiram-type reaction,
    metronidazole, 65
diuretics
  oedema, 54
  urea and electrolyte levels, 54
dopamine infusion
  calculations, 106, 109
  dose calculation, 109
  statements, 109
dopaminergic drugs, 33
dosing instructions, diazepam 5 mg
    tablets, 51
Dovonex ointment, side-effects, 30
doxycycline 100 mg capsules,
    cautionary labels, 27
doxycycline capsules, cautionary labels,
    72
drowsiness, drugs associated with, 74
drug interactions, 26, 67
  allopurinol, 26
  azathioprine, 26
  bendroflumethiazide, 26
  bisoprolol, 26
  carbamazepine, 26
  chlorpromazine, 26
  cimetidine tablets, 61
  digoxin, 57
  lithium, 26, 67
  methotrexate, 66
  simvastatin, 35
  St John's wort, 57
  theophylline, 26
  verapamil, 26, 35
drug interactions/cautions, 13
drug overdose, hypothermia, 19

drug-related seizures, drug monitoring,
    17
dry mouth, 33

E numbers
  butylated hydroxyanisole, 26
  glycerol, 26
  lecithin, 26
  names, 26
  ponceau 4R, 26
  sorbic acid, 9, 26
E45 cream, dose calculation, 111
ear infection
  Otomax (gentamicin compound), 48
  veterinary medicines, 48
eczema
  babies, 24
  Betnovate cream, 10
  Trimovate cream, 24
electrolyte imbalances
  digitalis toxicity, 20
  digoxin, 20, 47
  heart failure, 20
  lithium toxicity, 74
electrolyte levels, oedema, 54
electrolytes monitoring, renal
    impairment, 18
electronic cigarettes, smoking cessation,
    36
elixir volume, calculation, 93
emergency contraception
  acute porphyria, 17
  contraindicated drugs, 17
  course of action, 70
  emergency hormonal contraception
    (EHC), 40
  Levonelle, 17
  Levonelle One Step, 83
  statements, 83
  supplying, 40
emergency supply, 28–29, 64, 66
  atenolol, 64
  Logynon tablets, 84
  Microgynon, 45, 63
  nifedipine, 64
  oral contraceptive pills, 84
  qualifying healthcare professionals,
    63
  salbutamol inhaler, 84
  statements, 84

emetogenic chemotherapy drugs, 16
Emulsifying Ointment BP, calculation, 112–13
epilepsy treatment, 29
epilepsy, drugs to be avoided, 81
epinephrine (adrenaline), 28, 29
epinephrine (adrenaline), intramuscular
  anaphylactic reactions, 15
  children, 15
  dosage, 15
  nut allergy, 15
epoetin alfa, indications, 27
Eprex, 34
erectile dysfunction, sildenafil, 7, 56
errors
  lansoprazole, 85
  statements, 85
erythromycin 250 mg tablets, cautionary labels, 27
erythromycin capsules, dental prescription, 40
erythromycin coated tablets, cautionary labels, 79
estriol, calculation, 89
ethambutol, side-effects, 29
Eumovate cream, calculation, 95
expectorant drug, 75
eye infections, gonococcal
  licensed treatments, 24
  neonates, 24

fentanyl patches, calculation, 98
ferric complexes alternatives, parenteral feeding, 16
ferrous iron alternatives
  constipation, 12
  dosage, 12
fever, statements, 81
flu and cold remedies, 75
flu vaccinations
  asthma, 37
  children, 37
  HIV, 35–36
flucloxacillin
  cautionary labels, 73
  drug interactions, 82
  statements, 82
fluid replacement, syringe pump calculation, 115

fluoxetine, statements, 79
folate deficiency, side-effect, 29
folic acid, indications, 27
Fosamax, specific points, 23
FP10 prescriptions
  Cilest tablets, 8
  controlled drugs, 61
  Mefenamic acid tablets, 8
  number of NHS prescription charges, 8, 82
  requirements, 62
  sildenafil, 7
  Tranexamic acid tablets, 8
  warfarin, 8
fracture, atypical femoral
  drugs causing, 68
  knee pain, 68
furosemide
  side-effects, 73
  statements, 80
furosemide 40 mg OD
  dosage, 53
  oedema, 53
furosemide infusion, dilution calculation, 105

G6PD deficiency, haemolytic anaemia, 27–28
ganciclovir, 34
Gastrocote tablets, 31
general sales list (GSL) medicines
  over-the-counter (OTC) prescribing, 61
  statements, 83
generic names, reference sources, 54
gentamicin
  calculation, 92
  indications, 2
  Otomax (gentamicin compound), veterinary medicine, 48
  risks, 22
  side-effects, 2
  statements, 79
gentamicin intravenous infusion, statements, 80
gingival hyperplasia, drugs causing, 73–74
gliclazide, 27–28
  side-effects, 78
  statements, 78

glucagon, 27–28
glucose 12% solution, calculation, 91
glucose-6-phosphate dehydrogenase deficiency
    antibiotics prescribing, 8
    children, 8
    ethnic prevalence, 23
    haemolysis risk, 8, 23
    urinary-tract infection, 8
glycerol, E number, 26
gonococcal eye infections
    licensed treatments, 24
    neonates, 24
good dispensing practice, community pharmacy, 62–63
gout
    allopurinol, 66
    colchicine, 66
    drugs exacerbating, 24
    medicines precipitating, 54
GSL medicines. *See* general sales list medicines
Gynest cream, calculation, 89

H2-antagonists, 31
haemolysis risk
    antibiotics prescribing, 8
    children, 8
    glucose-6-phosphate dehydrogenase deficiency, 8, 23
    urinary-tract infection, 8
haemolytic anaemia
    drugs causing, 27–28
    G6PD deficiency, 27–28
half-life, calculation, 90
hay fever, 46
head lice
    statements, 87
    treatments, 87
headache, drugs treating, 85
heart failure
    beta-blockers, 69
    digitalis toxicity, 20
    digoxin, 20
    electrolyte imbalances, 20
heart toxicity, side-effect, 29
heparin, calculation, 100
hepatic encephalopathy, drugs treating, 76

HIV
    flu vaccinations, 35–36
    Zostavax vaccine, 35–36
homeopathy, 39
hormone replacement therapy (HRT), 6
    contraindicated conditions, 21
    hysterectomy patient, 18
    side-effects, 11
hydrocortisone 0.5% cream, prescribing quantities, 34
hydrocortisone 1% cream, over-the-counter (OTC) prescribing, 14
hydrocortisone cream
    calculation, 107
    counselling, 67
hydrocortisone tablets
    dosage, 10
    inflammatory condition, 10
    vs prednisolone tablets, 10
hypercalcaemia, drugs causing, 30
hypercholesterolaemia, simvastatin, 3
hyperglycaemia, 44
hyperkalaemia
    drugs causing, 30, 73
    statements, 82
hypermagnesaemia, drugs causing, 73
hypernatraemia, drugs causing, 30
hyperphosphataemia, drugs causing, 73
hypertension
    atorvastatin, 52
    first line treatment, 51
    lisinopril, 52
hypertensive crisis treatment, 29
hyperthyroidism
    drugs associated with, 74
    side-effect, 29
    sore throat, 46
hypoglycaemia
    drugs treating, 27–28
    renal impairment, 40
hypokalaemia, drugs causing, 30, 73
hyponatraemia
    drugs causing, 23, 30, 69
    statements, 33, 79
hypophosphataemia, drugs causing, 73
hypothermia, drug overdose, 19
hypothyroidism, drugs associated with, 74
hypromellose, calculation, 93

hysterectomy patient, hormone replacement therapy (HRT), 18

ibuprofen 5% gel, over-the-counter (OTC) prescribing, 14
ibuprofen, over-the-counter (OTC) prescribing, 61
infant formula products, prohibited promotion activities, 67
infection vulnerability, drugs causing, 77
inflammatory condition
hydrocortisone tablets, 10
prednisolone tablets, 10
influenza, vaccinations, 36, 37
infusion pump rate, calculation, 101
inhaler technique, drug used for improving, 30
INR (international normalised ratio), drugs causing an increase in, 57
insulin
calculation, 112
insulin types, identifying, 77
renal impairment, 40
intraocular pressure, 27
intrathecal administration, chemotherapy drugs, 15
intravenous additives, statements, 80
iodine, statements, 71
iron, 102, *See also* ferric complexes alternatives; ferrous iron alternatives, dose calculation
isoniazid
drug interactions, 79
statements, 79
isosorbide mononitrate, statements, 72
ispaghula, 28
itraconazole, dosage, 112
ivabradine, 31

Joint Formulary Committee, drug deemed less suitable for NHS prescribing, 30

Kabiven
magnesium ions concentration, 11
parenteral feeding, 11
kidney stones, 18, *See also* renal impairment, drugs causing

knee pain
drugs causing, 68
fracture, atypical femoral, 68

labelling. *See also* cautionary labels
clarithromycin 250 mg tablets, 27
doxycycline 100 mg capsules, 27
erythromycin 250 mg tablets, 27
legal requirements, 62
nifedipine, 64
nitrofurantoin 100 mg capsules, 27
Otomax (gentamicin compound), 48
oxytetracycline 250 mg tablets, 27
prescription accuracy checking, 49
'under the cascade', 17, 54
veterinary medicines, 17, 48, 54
labetolol, statements, 72
lansoprazole, errors, 85
Lantus injection, calculation, 112
Latin abbreviations used in prescribing, 21
lecithin, E number, 26
leflunomide
rheumatoid arthritis, 20
washout procedures, 20
legal requirements
labelling, 62
prescription legal requirements, morphine sulfate 10 mg/5mL oral solution, 70
legal restrictions on quantity sold, 75
Levonelle One Step, emergency contraception, 83
Levonelle, acute porphyria, 17
licensing, dexrazoxane, 21
lipoid pneumonia, drugs causing, 76
lisinopril
hypertension, 52
side-effects, 73
lithium
drug interactions, 26, 67, 82
Priadel (lithium carbonate), 30, 55
lithium toxicity
electrolyte imbalances, 74
signs/symptoms, 55
zopiclone, 55
liver failure, symptoms, 19
Logynon tablets, emergency supply, 84
loop diuretics, statements, 80
Lyclear Creme Rinse, statements, 87

Lyclear Dermal Cream
  body parts for application, 5
  maximum recommended usual
    quantity, 4
  scabies, 4–5

magnesium ions concentration
  Kabiven, 11
  parenteral feeding, 11
magnesium, statements, 71
malaria
  antimalarial medicines, pregnancy,
    87
  antimalarial medicines, statements,
    110
  Malarone tablets, calculation, 99
Malarone tablets, calculation, 99
male pattern baldness, drugs treating,
    76–77
mania prophylaxis/treatment, drugs
  used for, 73–74
Medicines Optimisation, 53
Medix Lifecare Nebuliser System, 30
Mefenamic acid tablets, FP10
  prescriptions, 8
menorrhagia, drugs treating symptoms
  of, 74
meropenem intravenous infusion, dose
  calculation, 109
metformin, 27–28
  diabetes, 55–56
  side-effects, 56
methotrexate
  advice, 4
  analgesics, concurrent, 4
  arthritis, 3–4
  conditions for caution, 3
  counselling, 4
  drug interactions, 66, 78
  side-effects, 29
  statements, 34
  toxicity signs, 4
metoclopramide
  nausea, 32
  pregnancy, 32
metoclopramide modified-release
  capsules, cautionary labels, 72
metronidazole
  disulfiram-type reaction, 65
  side-effects, 65

miconazole 2% cream, over-the-
  counter (OTC) prescribing, 14
Microgynon
  advice, 25
  emergency supply, 45, 63
  statements, 79
mifepristone, 33
minerals, statements, 71
Mini-Wright peak flow meter, 30
minocycline, cautionary labels, 73
MMR vaccine, contraindications, 5
morning after pill, 70, *See also*
  emergency contraception, course
  of action
morphine sulfate 10 mg/5mL oral
  solution, prescription legal
  requirements, 70
morphine sulfate, vs diamorphine
  subcutaneous infusion, 12
morphine, diamorphine. *See*
  diamorphine subcutaneous
  infusion
morphine, side-effects, 56
MST Continus 10mg tablets, 29
muscle spasm short-term relief, 29
myocardial infarction, acute
  cardiac enzymes and biomarkers, 25
  contraindicated drugs, 28
  diagnosing, 25
myocardial infarction, peptic ulcer,
    44–45

naproxen
  drug interactions, 80
  statements, 80
narcolepsy treatment, 29
nausea
  emetogenic chemotherapy drugs, 16
  metoclopramide, 32
  pregnancy, 32, 45
neonates. *See also* babies
  gonococcal eye infections, 24
  vancomycin, dose calculation, 116
neuropathic pain treatment, 29
New Medicines Service (NMS),
  statements, 68
NHS prescription charges
  FP10 prescriptions, number of NHS
    prescription charges, 8, 82

number of NHS prescription charges,
8, 82, 86
trigeminal neuralgia, 28
nicotine replacement products,
statements, 83
nifedipine
emergency supply, 64
labelling, 64
nitrofurantoin 100 mg capsules,
cautionary labels, 27
nitrofurantoin, urinary-tract infection,
8
NMS. *See* New Medicines Service
nut allergy
adrenaline (epinephrine),
intramuscular, 15
anaphylactic reactions, 15
children, 15
Nutrini® Multi Fibre Liquid,
statements, 114

octreotide, 28
oedema
diuretics, 53
electrolyte levels, 53
furosemide 40 mg OD, 53
urea and electrolyte levels, 53
olanzapine, 32
omeprazole, calculation, 91
opioids, conditions caused by long-term
use, 20
oral antibacterial therapy, cellulitis, 51
oral contraceptive pills
emergency supply, 84
statements, 79
oral typhoid vaccine, advice, 5
Oramorph, calculation, 97–98
osteoporosis, statements, 80
OTC prescribing. *See* over-the-counter
(OTC) prescribing
Otomax (gentamicin compound)
ear infection, 48
labelling, 48
veterinary medicines, 48
over-the-counter (OTC) prescribing, 61
clobetasone butyrate 0.05% cream,
14
diclofenac 2.32% gel, 14
general sales list (GSL) medicines, 61
hydrocortisone 1% cream, 14

ibuprofen, 61
ibuprofen 5% gel, 14
miconazole 2% cream, 14
overweight patients, antidiabetic
medications, 27–28
oxytetracycline 250 mg tablets,
cautionary labels, 27
oxytocin
effects, 22
risks, 22

P medicines. *See* pharmacy-only
medicines
pain
back pain, 6–7
knee pain, 68
neuropathic pain treatment, 29
postoperative anti-inflammatory,
children, 47
pain, chronic, morphine, 56
pain, moderate to severe, 27
palliative care
continuous subcutaneous infusions,
41
mixed drugs by syringe, 41
paracetamol
dosage, 35
dose calculation, 113
drug interactions, 82
paracetamol 120 mg/5 mL oral
suspension, children, 36–37
paraffin liquid, calculation, 111
paraffin, white soft
calculation, 112–13
dose calculation, 111
parenteral feeding. *See also* total
parenteral nutrition (TPN)
ferric complexes alternatives, 16
Kabiven, 11
magnesium ions concentration, 11
Parkinson's disease symptoms
alleviated by atropine eye drops,
69
patient care at risk, pharmacist's
behaviour and performance
concerns, 47
Patient Group Directives (PGDs)
statements, 19
supplying/administering under, 24
patient information disclosure, 67

patient medication record (PMR)
police access, 38
sore throat and fever, referral, 15
penicillamine, 33
penicillin allergy, drugs to be avoided,
75
penicillin V (phenoxymethylpenicillin),
cautionary labels, 73
Peptac liquid, 32
peptic ulcer
arthritis, 44–45
myocardial infarction, 44–45
proton pump inhibitors, 45
peripheral vascular disease treatment,
29
pertussis vaccine
children, 24
withholding, 24
pethidine, 32
PGDs. *See* Patient Group Directives
pharmacist's behaviour and
performance concerns, patient care
at risk, 47
pharmacy-only (P) medicines,
statements, 83
phenelzine, vs clomipramine, 13
phenoxymethylpenicillin 250 mg
tablets, private prescription
statements, 70
phenytoin
calculation, 98
continuity, 41
statements, 81
phosphorus, statements, 71
phototoxic reactions, drugs causing,
75
Piriton (chlorphenamine) syrup,
side-effects, 65
piroxicam
rheumatoid arthritis, 48
side-effects, 48
statements, 78
PMR. *See* patient medication record
Pocket Chamber, 30
police access, patient medication record
(PMR), 38
ponceau 4R, E number, 26
porphyria, acute. *See* acute porphyria
postoperative anti-inflammatory,
children, 47

potassium chloride
dose calculation, 105
side-effects, 29
potassium, statements, 82
prednisolone enteric-coated tablets,
calculation, 94
prednisolone tablets
calculation, 90
dosage, 10
inflammatory condition, 10
vs hydrocortisone tablets, 10
withdrawal, 20
prednisolone, dose calculation,
104–5
pregabalin, 29
pregnancy
analgesics, 6
antidiabetic medications, 22
antimalarial medicines, 87
back pain, 6–7
diabetes, 22
dinoprostone, contraindicated
circumstances, 23
labour induction, 23
metoclopramide, 32
mifepristone, 33
nausea, 32, 45
premature labour inhibition, 27–28
spina bifida prevention, 27
teratogenic drugs, 21
premature labour inhibition, drugs used
for, 27–28
premises, statements, 83
prescribing
drug deemed less suitable for NHS
prescribing, 30
drug prohibited for NHS prescribing,
30
Joint Formulary Committee, 30
prescription accuracy checking, 49
prescription charges, NHS. *See* NHS
prescription charges
prescription date, temazepam tablets,
50
prescription legal requirements,
morphine sulfate 10 mg/5mL oral
solution, 70
prescription statements,
phenoxymethylpenicillin 250 mg
tablets, 70

Index **197**

prescriptions, computer-generated, statements, 70
Priadel (lithium carbonate)
  side-effects, 30, 55
  toxicity, 30, 55
privacy, statements, 83
prohibited for NHS prescribing, drug, 30
propranolol
  asthma, 57
  contraindications, 57
  diabetes, 57
  statements, 78, 80
protease, calculation, 112
proton pump inhibitors, peptic ulcer, 45
pseudoephedrine, statements, 72–73
pulmonary fibrosis, drugs associated with, 74

QT intervals, drugs associated with prolonged, 22

ramipril alternatives for dry cough, 10
ramipril, statements, 72
red urine, drugs causing, 76
referral, patient medication record (PMR), sore throat and fever, 15
refrigeration temperature, recommended, 55
renal function, calculation, 96
renal impairment
  anaemia associated with chronic renal failure, 27
  drugs to be avoided, 24
  electrolytes monitoring, 18
  hypoglycaemia, 40
  insulin, 40
repeat prescriptions
  amlodipine, 2–3
  aspirin, 2–3
  simvastatin, 2–3
  statin therapy, 2–3
respiratory symptoms monitoring, 30
returned medicines, good dispensing practice, 63
Reye's syndrome, drugs associated with, 74
rheumatoid arthritis
  anti-rheumatic drugs, 20

counselling, 43–44
depression, 48
leflunomide washout procedures, 20
piroxicam, 48
urinary-tract infection, 43–44
Rifater tablets, calculation, 92
Rifinah capsules, dose calculation, 109

salbutamol, 27–28
salbutamol inhaler
  asthma, 59–60, 84
  emergency supply, 84
  side-effects, 60
  statements, 84
  techniques, 60
salbutamol syrup, asthma, 60
salicylic acid cream, calculation, 107
scabies
  dermatological preparations, 4–5
  Lyclear Dermal Cream, 4–5
schedule 1 controlled drugs, 29
schedule 2 controlled drugs, 61
schedules, controlled drugs, 51
schizophrenia,
  clozapine/chlorpromazine dose equivalence, 9
seizures
  drug-related seizures, drug monitoring, 17
  drugs exacerbating, 73–74
side-effects
  amiloride, 73
  amiodarone, 29
  amitriptyline, 56
  amlodipine, 64
  antipsychotics, 20
  beclometasone 100 mcg inhaler, 64
  bendroflumethiazide, 73
  Bricanyl respules 5 mg/2mL, 30
  Buscopan (hyoscine butylbromide) tablets, 61
  chlorphenamine (Piriton) syrup, 65
  colour vision disturbance, 29
  constipation, 29
  corticosteroids, 23
  Desmotabs 200 mcg tablets, 30
  Dovonex ointment, 30
  dry eyes, 28
  ethambutol, 29
  folate deficiency, 29

side-effects (*continued*)
furosemide, 73
gentamicin, 2
gliclazide, 78
heart toxicity, 29
hormone replacement therapy
  (HRT), 11
hypercalcaemia, 30
hyperkalaemia, 30, 73
hypermagnesaemia, 73
hypernatraemia, 30
hyperphosphataemia, 73
hyperthyroidism, 29
hypokalaemia, 30, 73
hyponatraemia, 30
hypophosphataemia, 73
lisinopril, 73
metformin, 55–56
methotrexate, 29
metronidazole, 65
morphine, 56
Piriton (chlorphenamine) syrup,
  65
piroxicam, 48
potassium chloride, 29
Priadel (lithium carbonate), 30,
  55
salbutamol inhaler, 59–60
simvastatin, 3
spironolactone 50 mg tablets, 30
Trimovate cream, 24
weight gain, 20
sildenafil
children, 40
diabetes, 7, 56
erectile dysfunction, 7, 56
FP10 prescriptions, 7
mode of action, 40
prescription endorsement, 7, 56
simvastatin, 28
dosage, 2–3
drug interactions, 35
hypercholesterolaemia, 2–3
monitoring, 2–3
repeat prescriptions, 2–3
side-effects, 2–3
smoking cessation
asthma, 84
electronic cigarettes, 36
salbutamol inhaler, 84

sodium bicarbonate 4.2% intravenous
  infusion, dilution calculation,
  115
sodium chloride aqueous solution,
  calculation, 112
sodium chloride in isotonic solution,
  33
sodium levels
calculation, 108
statements, 79
sodium nitroprusside, 29
sorbic acid
allergy, 9
E number, 26, 9
sore throat
advice, 46
hyperthyroidism, 46
sore throat and fever, referral, 15
spina bifida prevention, 27
spironolactone 50 mg tablets,
  side-effects, 30
St John's wort, 34
digoxin, 57
drug interactions, 57
staphylococcal skin infection
acute porphyria, 1–2
antibiotics prescribing, 1–2
children, 1–2
statin therapy. *See also* atorvastatin;
  simvastatin
monitoring, 3
repeat prescriptions, 3
statements, 79
sterilisation methods, 50
steroid inhalers, statements, 82
stomach ulcer, drugs causing, 66
strontium ranelate, contraindicated
  patients, 21
Sudafed tablets, 30
sumatriptan, 40
syringe drivers, compatibility of drugs,
  18

tardive dyskinesia, drugs causing,
  73
teeth staining, drugs causing, 76
Tegaderm hydrocolloid dressings,
  adverse reactions, 87
telephoning patients, good dispensing
  practice, 63